ADVANCE PRAISE

"The Science of a Long Life affirms not only knowledge Dr. Fuster has about the human body and aging but also his compassion and practicality for all of us. I would do whatever he tells me to do in this book to live a long and healthy life."

BOB HARPER, HOST OF THE BIGGEST
LOSER AND BEST-SELLING AUTHOR

"When I first met Dr. Valentin Fuster, it was to interview him about a study he had just published using beta-blockers in a way that had previously been thought to be contraindicated in heart failure. That was my first exposure to Valentin Fuster's approach to medicine: challenge the status quo, question conventional thinking, and demand evidence. That tactic has enabled Dr. Fuster to advance the science of cardiology in ways that have saved countless lives. Now he is applying it to something we are all interested in: living a longer and healthier life.

As a medical journalist for nearly four decades, I have had the privilege of observing and reporting on breathtaking advances in medicine. But it is the last few years that have brought us to what former vice-president Joseph Biden called an inflection point in medicine's ability to treat and even cure many of humankind's most difficult afflictions.

It is those scientific developments that are being applied to the field of antiaging that Dr. Fuster and Josep Corbella so clearly and engagingly describe in this book. Yes, we should all have reason to believe that age truly is just a number. From genetics and antiaging molecules to stem cells, exercise, sex, and wrinkles, The Science of a Long Life gives us the guide we need to expand our life span and, more importantly, our health span. Thank you, Valentin. I feel younger already!"

DR. MAX GOMEZ, WCBS MEDICAL REPORTER

"To have been asked to comment on my dear friend Dr. Valentin Fuster's The Science of a Long Life is not only an honor for me but also a great opportunity to share some ideas that I firmly believe in: a strict discipline, a strong will, perseverance, enthusiasm, and a positive mind. My motto has always been, "If I rest, I rust." These are not simply words; they are facts. My most sincere congratulations to Dr. Fuster for this book and for the gift that it represents when a man of his knowledge tells us that "to surrender is not an option."

PLÁCIDO DOMINGO, SINGER, CONDUCTOR,
ELI AND EDYTHE BROAD GENERAL
DIRECTOR OF LOS ANGELES OPERA

"Dr. Valentin Fuster has worked for decades to create substantial and enduring bonds with scientists and health organizations around the world to address disparities that exist in cardiovascular disease risk factors, awareness, and life expectancy. Dr. Fuster's tireless and steadfast dedication to science has significantly advanced research discoveries and clinical care internationally."

NANCY BROWN, CEO, AMERICAN HEART ASSOCIATION

"Valentin Fuster is one of the most accomplished physicians in the world. He is a man of high character and a role model for generations of physicians and scientists. There is no one better to guide us toward a long life of achievement and joy."

DR. DENNIS S. CHARNEY, ANNE AND JOEL EHRENKRANZ DEAN, ICAHN SCHOOL OF MEDICINE AT MOUNT SINAI

THE SCIENCE OF A LONG LIFE

THE
SCIENCE
OF A
LONG LIFE

DR. VALENTIN FUSTER
JOSEP CORBELLA

THE SCIENCE OF A LONG LIFE
The Art of Living More and the Science of Living Better

ISBN   978-1-5445-0103-1 *Paperback*

978-1-5445-0102-4 *Ebook*

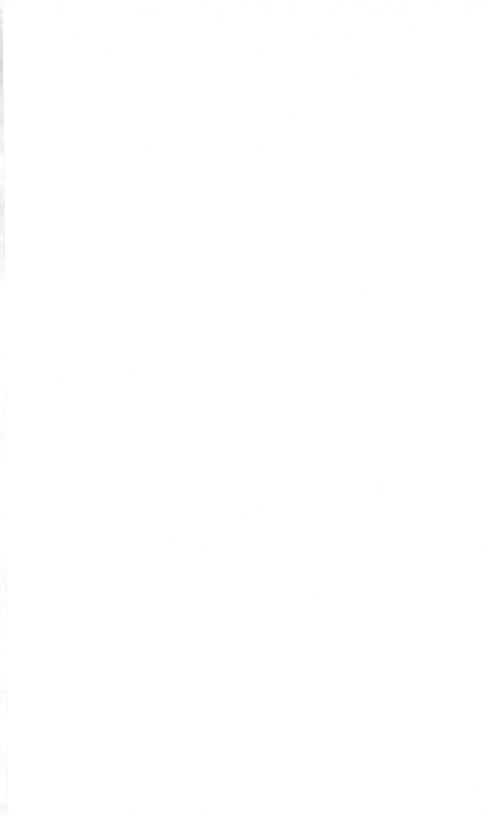

CONTENTS

FOREWORD BY RAFAEL NADAL

Dispelling your doubts, time and again.

For those of us who have been playing professional sports for a long time, we always have to continue to dispel the rumors about our retirement. Not many people expected to see me competing at "my" level after I turned thirty. Not a very ancient age for a sport such as tennis, although it has to be said that I've been a professional since 2001— by coincidence the year when Pau made his debut in the NBA—and since 2003 in the Top 100.

Throughout my career, some predicted that I wouldn't last long—that I wouldn't even play for ten years. Sporting longevity for someone who had started young is a prize. We age quicker because we expose our bodies to the highest possible level of physical demands to yield spectacular results.

We athletes are extreme cases of willpower and perseverance. Pau is an excellent example of this. We're both very strict and disciplined. But I think that everyone, even those without extraordinary physical aptitude, can lead a healthy life for many years.

Valentín Fuster and Josep Corbella show us in their book that the mental dimension is as important as the physical aspect of slowing down the process of aging. Without willpower, your body won't obey you. And without the body's cooperation, it's time to take a break, recover, and check if the willpower and enthusiasm are still there. Are they? Let's go. Let's give it our all once more. Return and return, and win and win.

Each individual has their own way of facing the passage of time. I need rhythm, demands, hard training. This gives me the confidence to compete in tournaments. I know perfectly well what's good and bad for me. I think I know the secret to a long sporting life, and that if I feel well and happy, this will help me have a long life outside of sports.

Many people think that we live obsessed with our sport. And while it's true that sometimes it can reach that level, it's not always the case. Sporting life, no matter how intense and exceptional it is, isn't your entire life. I have no idea when I'll retire. I haven't got any specific plans. I think most of us don't think about these things until the decision is made. We athletes are "old young people," facing situations and decisions that usually come much later in life for most people. When I stop having fun playing, I'll do other things that excite me, such as my Tennis Academy that is already operational.

Finding your purpose and happiness in life is nearly everything you need. That's what Fuster and Corbella write about. This helps your odds for having a long life. Dr. Fuster, at seventy-four, preaches his own example. He's more active than ever. His lust for life is contagious. His example inspires us. I recommend following him and reading what he has to say.

FOREWORD BY PAU GASOL

Age is just a number.

This is how Valentín Fuster and Josep Corbella start this magnificent book. And basketball is a sport of numbers, statistics, averages, and records. In this sea of data, age always tends to stick out. Due to the requirement level of the NBA—the frequency of the games, their intensity, game minutes, constant travel, the competition—the time players spend in the league is usually shorter than in other sports. Players who are still playing at forty are rare exceptions. In fact, only three are still active in the 2017/2018 season, and only twenty players are over thirty-five. Some are called "grandads."

This is the destiny of professional athletes: promise before twenty, maturity around the age of thirty, and "grandad" at forty. Age is no more than a perception.

In this book you are about to read, full of wisdom based on scientific studies, you will learn different factors that will help you lead a better-quality life.

Milestones are measured according to age. All too often, we see statistics related to the duration of your life. By late 2017, I had become the first player over thirty-seven to score at least fourteen points, ten rebounds, and five assists in four games in a row. Numbers, data adorning a service page—but just accessories if by the end of the fourth quarter your team hasn't won the game. The titles trumpeted that this was "despite my age" and that I was going through a "second youth."

At thirty-seven and with over 40,000 minutes of play in seventeen seasons, I'm the ninth most senior player of the league. According to NBA average statistics, I should have retired a few years ago. But here I am, still. With the years comes the benefit of experience and an intimate knowledge of your own capabilities, so that your highs are never too high, and your lows are never too low.

Yes, Fuster and Corbella are right: age is just a number if you frame it that way for yourself. Aging isn't a problem. For me, one of the key takeaways from the book that speaks to me most is the concept of "ikigai." For those of you who don't know it, I will leave for you to discover further on.

We professional athletes age faster. Rafa and I know this well. Our organisms are subjected to blows and pressures—constant changes that wear us down much quicker than others. Our joints are subjected to repeated movements involving great forces and loads, because repetition is the only way of achieving excellence: one shot, a step back, a free throw...Your body suffers, the recovery process becomes longer, and as you age, you need more time, more discipline, and—it also has to be said—more sacrifice. Add to this tally the injuries, the months of recovery, and the preparations, and without specific treatments and preparations, no professional could hope to play ten, fifteen, or twenty years.

One of the secrets of a long life in sports is the work you do to strengthen yourself and prevent injuries—something I've focused a lot on with my medical team. But obviously injuries happen, and you need the mental and emotional capability to overcome these bumps in the road, together with the willpower and drive necessary to return to the point you were at before, or even better. On this subject, Rafael Nadal has a long track record of fantastic returns.

Naturally, this is my profession and my passion. I'm

dedicated to it in the literal sense of the word. I've fully accepted the effort and pain that go with it, and I have no regrets—quite the contrary. Taking care of myself is not an option; it's a professional obligation to keep performing at my level. My best investment has been in myself, keeping up my performance level, thanks to the incredible professionals who have helped me and continue to do so.

Longevity fascinates us because it holds secrets—whether it's a person at one hundred years of age or a professional athlete about to turn forty or playing for over fifteen years. This book has compiled the secrets that are within anyone's reach. They don't entail large investments, but they do require willpower and a strong conviction. These secrets are revealed by two top athletes.

Valentín Fuster, whom I know better out of the two, is a close friend of mine. He knows and understands athletes well. We have many things in common. A deep-seated love for sports, to name just one thing. Perhaps many of you didn't know that Dr. Fuster climbs the Col du Tourmalet every year and that, when he was a teenager, he wanted to be a professional tennis player.

We also share a passion for medicine: if I hadn't become a professional basketball player, I'd have continued my medical studies at the Bellvitge Campus of the University of Barcelona and, knowing me, today I'd be proud to be a good doctor. Dr. Fuster doesn't only work in medicine, but he makes it into something friendly, as well. His work isn't as flamboyant as that of an athlete. There are no cameras filming and no journalists at the exit from the operating room asking his opinion about the operation. Nevertheless, without trying to compare professions, I can't think of a more valuable and transcendent career than that of saving and/or prolonging life.

We share common roots—Catalan and Spanish—and the fact we both started an American adventure, and both living our professional dream. We also have a grand goal in common: we want to have a real impact on people's lives. Well aware of this, we've decided to work together, sharing health habits that prevent child obesity and cardiovascular disease—two illnesses with much in common. We've joined forces, together with our foundations, and we're both trying to contribute the best from our specialties: his experience in health care and my sporting track record.

I'm sure that, with this book, readers will endorse some habits and knowledge that will bring them long-term benefits, if applied correctly. There are many to choose from—check them out. The science of a long life can be put to practice regardless of your age. Here, we give you the blueprint. All you need to do is follow the steps. And take ownership of your goals.

AGE IS JUST A NUMBER

WE CAN'T CHANGE OUR CHRONOLOGICAL AGE, BUT WE CAN CHANGE OUR BIOLOGICAL AGE

It's one of the most common questions between people who have just met. Adults ask it when they want to initiate a conversation with a child. Airlines ask it when selling tickets online. Insurance companies, when we buy an insurance policy. A doctor, when seeing his patient for the first time.

The first question is usually the name, and then comes age. If it is such a common question, it is because it provides useful information. Twenty-four years old? Too young to run the company. Sixty-five years old? Too old for new ideas. Thirty-eight years old? Could be my girlfriend!

If one stops to think about why this small bit of information is so useful, it is because our brain prefers simplicity. We like to think we have been graced with the most complex organ in the universe, that we are intelligent creatures—so much so that we have not hesitated to call ourselves *Homo sapiens* (which, by the way, is a self-description). However, if we are being honest, we must admit that complexity makes us uncomfortable. We are not as *sapiens* as we would like to think; we try to simplify things when given the chance; and we fall into the temptation of generalizing.

This has its advantages. Dividing the world, and the rest of humanity, into categories allows us to make quick decisions that most times are accurate. Consider a doctor, for example. If you are a woman over fifty, a mammogram is recommended. If your blood pressure is higher than 140, it is classified as hypertension. If you weigh 264 pounds and are 5'6" tall, you will be classified as obese. Doctors are not the only ones to do it, of course. We all do it. If a student gets nothing but top marks in math, we label him or her as intelligent. If they get nothing but low marks, we may not say anything, but inwardly, we label them as well. We divide the world into boxes, each with its appropriate label, and that makes our life easier.

But this very human habit of labeling everything has its drawbacks. Is a twenty-four-year-old person too young to run a company? Look at Mark Zuckerberg, who had already founded Facebook by the age of twenty. A sixty-five-year-old man can no longer learn new ideas? Picasso continued to paint and experiment well into his nineties. And let us not forget Pope Francis, who is revolutionizing the Catholic Church after having been elected at the age of seventy-six.

Zuckerberg, Picasso, and the Pope are exceptional cases, but the tendency to generalize affects us all. It is a very common practice that can make us fall back on prejudices and make mistakes. Not so long ago in Europe and North America, black people were regarded to be of inferior intelligence to whites. Women were considered unfit to vote, or more recently, were considered less able than men at math. There are some who still think that way, and they are wrong.

Today, we know that such discriminations have no scientific basis and are the result of prejudice and ignorance. But they do invite us to ask ourselves which stereotypes we have today that we unquestioningly accept as normal (such as when it was considered normal to consider women unfit to vote), will be judged unfounded and unfair in the future.

IS A TWENTY-FOUR-YEAR-OLD PERSON REALLY TOO YOUNG TO RUN A COMPANY? LOOK AT MARK ZUCKERBERG, WHO HAD ALREADY FOUNDED FACEBOOK BY THE AGE OF TWENTY. A SIXTY-FIVE-YEAR-OLD MAN CAN NO LONGER LEARN NEW IDEAS? PICASSO CONTINUED TO PAINT AND EXPERIMENT WELL INTO HIS NINETIES. AND POPE FRANCIS IS REVOLUTIONIZING THE CHURCH AFTER BEING ELECTED AT THE AGE OF SEVENTY-SIX.

Think, for example, about the attitudes we have regarding age—both our own as well as others'. We encourage young children to define themselves by their age. From the perspective of a four-year-old boy, a child who is five is older and one who is three is younger. He is constantly asked his age and is taught to celebrate the change of age with cakes and gifts.

Birthdays, as we know, are a cause for celebration, until they are not anymore. One day, we realize that happy birthday has become a not-so-happy birthday, and instead of turning one year older, we would rather turn a year younger. In private, we might allow ourselves to celebrate, but in public, many of us opt for discretion, isn't that so?

We all know that this is absurd, that being forty-five years and a day old is not very different from being forty-five years and a day younger. Nor is it very different to be forty than it is to be thirty-nine. However, we speak of the midlife crisis at forty, fifty, even at sixty. And these crises really exist. They do not affect everyone equally, but there are many people who experience them, and data from multiple studies support this.

When researchers from New York University and UCLA (University of California, Los Angeles) analyzed the age of first-time marathon runners, the largest number were runners of an age ending in nine. Respectively, twenty-nine, thirty-nine, forty-nine, and fifty-nine years of age represented 14.8 percent of all those registered, instead of the 10 percent that would be expected if they did not have that additional motivation. Ages ending in nine are the ages that make you aware you are entering a new decade and feel that you are getting older.

When analyzing the times of amateur marathon runners, the best records also belong to those of an age ending in nine. On average, they run 2.3 percent faster than athletes of other ages. Their "milestone" ages explain why these athletes are more motivated and probably better prepared for the race.

The same pattern, even more pronounced, can be observed when analyzing the age of married men seeking extra-marital relationships on dating sites. Of those registered,

17.9 percent are of an age ending in nine, instead of the expected 10 percent. The search for an extramarital relationship is considered an indication—although this cannot be proven empirically—that a person is going through an existential crisis and seeks to add more meaning to their life.

All of this is somewhat absurd, even comical. These are small scenes within the great human comedy. Why worry so much about turning a decade older? Just because nature has equipped us with five fingers on each hand and we learned to count by tens? If we had only four fingers, we would have an age crisis every eight years, which would be even more uncomfortable. If we had six fingers, we would be lucky to be able to count in twelves. But we have five fingers, and we worship the decimal system and, more generally, numbers. Our brain has a natural inclination to count, measure, and classify. We count pounds, degrees, cholesterol, times, distances, calories, prices, goals...and naturally, years as well. Everything that can be counted.

The problem is that years do not truly tell us how much younger or older we are. All they tell us is how many years have passed since we were born—what we might call our chronological age. But being younger or older—what we could call our biological age—is, like everything else related to the human body, more complex and subtle.

We have all seen that some people age more slowly than others. There are those who seem old at seventy-seven and those who seem relatively young at eighty. Young due to their health, because they feel good and stay active, but also due to their attitude, because they have projects and have not lost their desire to accomplish their goals.

A clear proof that chronological age does not necessarily correspond with biological age is that longevity runs in families. In some households, it is normal to live past ninety years of age. In others, household members will be hard-pressed to remember anyone living past eighty-five.

In the Greek island of Ikaria, where life expectancy is ten years greater than in the rest of Europe, a third of the population lives longer than ninety years. In the Japanese island of Okinawa, the likelihood of reaching a hundred is three times higher than in the rest of Japan. There must be something special about the inhabitants of these islands that explains their exceptional longevity.

Further evidence of the difference between chronological age and biological age is that in almost all cultures of the world, life expectancy for women is higher than men. Due to some of the many differences between the female body and the male body, women age a little more slowly.

At this point, an inevitable question arises: if chronological age is less important, how can we know what our biological age is?

The US Center for Disease Control and Prevention has created a formula for calculating the heart age of a person, starting with their chronological age and adjusting it according to sex, blood pressure, smoking habits, diabetes, and body mass index (a measure of body fat based on your weight in relation to your height). This initiative has the virtue of showing that, if we take care of ourselves, we can prevent premature cardiac aging. But the downside is that it does not really clarify our biological age, because aging is a process that affects the entire body, not just the heart.

A test has also been developed to calculate biological age based on the length of the telomeres in white blood cells. Telomeres are DNA fragments that shorten with aging, which we will explain in more detail in chapter 3. For now, suffice it to say that given that telomeres become shorter throughout our lifespan, their length can be considered a marker of biological age. But again, aging does not affect only telomeres.

A research team from Duke University in North Carolina has gone a step further and devised a system to calculate biological age based on data spanning the entire body. They have assessed the state of the cardiovascular system, the immune system, the liver, the kidneys, the lungs, the gums, the arteries of the retina, the integrity of the DNA...They have done tests to measure intellectual performance and physical agility. They have considered what age each person might seem based on appearance, which was assessed by observers who did not know the person's actual chronological age. In summary, it is a complete package.

The Duke researchers input all this data into computers and then implemented an algorithm to calculate the biological age of each person. Not surprisingly, this system is very expensive and impractical. Few people will be willing to go through so many tests just to find out what an algorithm has to say about his or her alleged biological age. But the results of the investigation are revealing.

When this algorithm was applied to a group of 954 men and women born thirty-eight years prior, it was observed that only 20 percent had a biological age of thirty-eight. For the vast majority, the biological age was distributed between thirty-four and forty-two years of age. This means that the biological age differed from the chronological age up to 10 percent, either above or below. This was true for the vast majority.

There was also a small minority of lucky people who did not even reach the biological age of thirty. This means that they showed a rejuvenation of more than 20 percent compared to their chronological age. Another small minority had aged prematurely and had the health equivalent of someone over fifty.

An interesting fact is that the physical appearance of the participants in the study, which had not undergone any cosmetic treatments, accurately reflected each participant's biological age. Meaning, those who appeared to be thirty years old had a biological age of around thirty years old. Those who seemed to be forty had the biology of someone who was forty. This means that the body performed as if it were forty years old.

What is most interesting is that, although we cannot do anything to change our chronological age, we can change the biological age. At least to a certain extent, because aging faster or slower depends largely on our genes. Thus, longevity does run in families. But it also depends largely on how well we care for or mistreat our bodies and what we do with them, not only physically but also emotionally and intellectually. It depends on our behavior but also on our attitude. Basically, we decide how we live.

Participants of research studies at Duke University were also analyzed for a span of twelve years, from ages twenty-six to thirty-eight. It was noted that some had aged more rapidly and others more slowly. All of them considered themselves young. When asked their age, they would say thirty-eight. But some were aging at full speed. What lesson can we draw from this? Simply that if we want to stay younger longer and have a long life and enjoy it, the sooner we start to care for ourselves, the better the results we'll see.

When you think about it, research on longevity—how to add years to life and life to years—has traditionally focused on older people. Which is fine, but if younger people were also taken into account, it would be even better. Growing old is like a woodworm. It does not begin later in life, but rather when growth stops happening. It advances stealthily through the years. And when we finally realize it is there, much of the damage has been done.

> Growing old is like a woodworm. It does not begin later in life, but rather the moment growth stops. It advances stealthily through the years. And when we finally realize it is there, much of the damage is already done.

You may have noticed that none of the methods for measuring biological age are satisfactory. We have no way of knowing the exact age of our cells, tissues, and organs. You can view it as testament to our ignorance: how little we truly know about growing older and how much science has yet to learn. If you expected this book to hold all the answers, return it now and ask for your money back!

In essence, we are lucky that we cannot really find out our

biological age. More than likely, there will come a day not too far in the future where more reliable biological age tests will be offered. We will either get good news ("You are eight years younger than what your ID says.") or useful information to improve our health ("You are eight or more years older; let's see what we can do to help."). If we look at it the other way around, it could be said that these tests provide us with bad news or useless information.

Will we live better when we have these tests, or will we simply replace discrimination based on chronological age with a new discrimination based on biological age? With this information, an insurance company could accept or reject a client. A company in countries where there are no laws to prohibit it could decide whether or not to hire an employee. A dating website could segregate its users...The possibilities for discrimination are endless, and almost all of them infringe on individual liberties.

Ultimately, what does growing old mean? It is not the exact same thing as turning a year older. It is easily confused because it is two processes that move forward with time. Years are measured with a number, objective and unquestionable, and they determine what others think of us. But the most important thing in growing old is how we see ourselves. It is a process of vulnerability—physical as well as mental—that cannot be reduced to a number. Of course, some of the aging parameters can be measured objectively, such as the decline of our respiratory capacity, the loss of hearing or vision, or the number of drugs we take. Other parameters are subjective: the feeling of being capable of doing things, the desire to do those things, and the capacity to enjoy each and every day. These are the most important, and there is no test that can measure them.

Chronological Age, Misleading Appearance

For most people, biological age does not correspond to chronological age

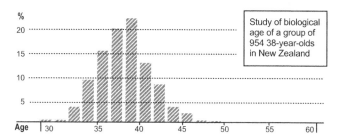

Study of biological age of a group of 954 38-year-olds in New Zealand

What we believe...
At what age is a person considered to begin aging?

Age you consider old age begins

Real age	
18-29	60
30-49	69
50-64	72
65 or more	74

...and what we experience
How do you feel in regard to your age?

Young Same age Old Didn't know/Didn't answer

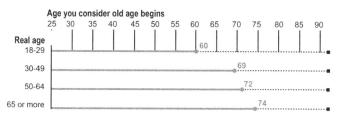

Age: 18-29, 30-49, 50-64, 65-74, 75 or more

Fuentes: PNAS / *The Wall Street Journal*

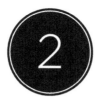

WRINKLES

THE MOST OBVIOUS CHANGES
ARE NOT THE MOST IMPORTANT

The mirror, wrote Borges, is abhorrent because it duplicates a person. What he did not write, but probably thought, is that every day it duplicates a person differently from the previous day. We've all experienced this transformation. We bring the mirror close to our face and find a spot that was not there yesterday, a wrinkle that has become deeper, a random gray hair...The changes that come with age become more evident as they accumulate. The more changes there are, the more difficult it is to ignore them. And there is no part of the body where change is more evident than the skin. The mirror makes sure we remember this every morning.

The changes that occur in the skin are not very different

from those stealthily taking place inside the body. They are different in appearance, because wrinkles, gray hair, and blemishes are unique to the tissues of the skin. But in essence, they are similar, for all tissues tend to degrade through the same processes. So understanding how skin ages and what can be done to stop its deterioration can teach us how to understand and curb the aging process throughout the body.

No one, no matter how much they try, can maintain youthful-looking skin at an advanced age. After the age of twenty, the amount of collagen that gives skin its firmness begins to decrease. Collagen is the most abundant protein in the human body, and it is responsible for maintaining the integrity of fibrous tissues such as muscles, tendons, ligaments, and cartilages. It acts as a flexible mold—a kind of frame that gives tissues their shape.

In the skin, the amount of collagen decreases at a rate of about 1 percent each year. If the decline begins at twenty years of age, once we reach forty, the collagen in our skin has reduced by about 28 percent. By the time we are sixty, 32 percent. And, with the decrease in collagen, it is not surprising that the appearance of the skin changes with age. It becomes more flaccid.

Over the years, there is also a reduction in the amount of elastin, a protein that gives elasticity to the skin and other tissues, as its name suggests. By simply pressing someone's forearm with a fingernail, we can understand what elastin does. On a younger person's skin, the mark left by the fingernail will vanish quickly, but older skin will take longer to regain its initial form. The older we get, the longer it takes. It is not serious, nor a flaw, nor anything to be ashamed of. It is simply that older people have less elastin.

There is a third component of the skin that declines with age. I am referring to—you might want to take a breath before saying this—glycosaminoglycans, or GAGs, if you prefer the acronym. They are molecules that abound in the human body and attract water. They are said to be hydrophilic. You have probably heard of some of them. If you have ever had a knee injury and had hyaluronic acid injected into it, know those are GAGs improving the lubrication of the joint. In the skin, the GAGs are in charge of good hydration. But as the skin gradually loses its ability to produce GAGs, it becomes drier and more brittle with age.

NO ONE, NO MATTER HOW CAREFUL, CAN MAINTAIN YOUTHFUL-LOOKING SKIN AT AN ADVANCED AGE. AFTER THE AGE OF TWENTY, THE AMOUNT OF COLLAGEN THAT OUR SKIN PRODUCES BEGINS TO DECREASE. IT ACTS AS A FLEXIBLE MOLD—A KIND OF FRAME THAT HOLDS THE TISSUES.

To all of this, we add the redistribution of fat. In a young face, fat found directly under the skin (or subcutaneous fat) is distributed uniformly, which gives it the soft round shape we associate with beauty. In older people, the volume of subcutaneous fat is reduced and the face becomes more angular. At the same time, fat tends to move downward due to gravity; bags under the eyes may appear, as well as sagging cheeks or jowls.

These are all changes that dermatologists call intrinsic, because they come from inside the body. But they are not the only factors influencing skin aging. There are also changes caused by bad treatment of the skin, called extrinsic by dermatologists because they come from external aggressions.

The most common aggression on your skin, which you have probably already heard of, is solar radiation. A little sun is desirable, even essential. If we are never exposed to the sun, we lack vitamin D, which occurs naturally in the skin and is necessary for its proper formation and maintenance. The sun also has positive psychological effects. During autumn, when days become shorter and gray, some people feel sadder because they lack the joy caused by sunlight.

However, too much sun has more disadvantages than advantages, at least for the skin. Ultraviolet rays are to blame, causing a degradation of not only aesthetics, but also function.

We have special skin cells that produce melanin in response to ultraviolet radiation. Melanin is the pigment that makes us brown, which acts as a protective shield and which our society considers attractive. But in order to achieve this attractive protection, we must pay a high price.

The problem is that ultraviolet rays are more energetic than visible light and have destructive capacities. One of the skin's victims is cell DNA, which suffers genetic mutations when exposed to ultraviolet radiation. The more radiation, the more mutations. That is why too much sun increases the risk of skin cancer.

The other two victims are collagen and elastin, the two proteins that give the skin a youthful appearance. Collagen decreases with ultraviolet radiation, even without getting sunburned. And elastin forms clusters of irregular fibers that alter the appearance of the skin and cause what dermatologists call solar elastosis. It is what gives people who have spent thousands of hours exposed to sun, such as sailors or farmers, that leathery-looking skin.

Next we have damage caused by tobacco, which is the second most common extrinsic aggression to the skin. There are cases where an observant person can tell if someone is a smoker or not simply by their appearance, at least if they are heavy smokers. There is even a clinical term called "smoker face." It is characterized by premature wrinkles, especially around the eyes in the form of crow's feet and around the lips, and as changes in texture and color of the skin that give the face a haggard aspect. It affects 8 percent of people who have smoked for ten years, and the percentage increases the longer the person has been smoking.

It is not known exactly how tobacco causes this accelerated aging of the skin. We know that the presence of smoke in the air dries the skin from outside the body; that on the inside, toxic tobacco byproducts reach the skin through the blood; that these toxic molecules provoke inflammation of which the smoker is unaware; and that the inflammation alters the skin's appearance. This in turn causes the secretion of enzymes called metalloproteins (or MMP). The MMP—which, by the way, also occur in response to the sun's ultraviolet rays—decrease collagen. With the decrease of collagen, as previously explained, the skin loses firmness and the appearance of wrinkles is accelerated. However, this is probably not the complete story; there are other ways tobacco damages the skin that have not yet been discovered.

In any case, the two examples of ultraviolet rays and tobacco are enough to illustrate the important issue at hand. As previously explained, in relation to the skin and any other tissue, aging has intrinsic causes derived from the simple fact of being alive. If we live, we age. There is no alternative to this universal law. But aging is also modulated by external factors that depend on how we choose to live. It depends on whether we benefit from the sun or burn our skin. It depends on whether we smoke or not.

These external factors, as we have seen, act upon intrinsic causes and regulate them. If we accumulate MMP, we damage our collagen. If we abuse our bodies with radiations, toxins, and other aggressions, we speed up the aging process. However, in the same way we can accelerate it, we can also stop it. In the following pages and chapters, we will see how.

In the case of the skin, the first things that come to mind when we talk about stopping the aging process are aesthetic medical treatments. Facelifts, Botox, fillers, creams... Few areas in medicine have increased their activity in recent decades, built as many clinics, and made as much money as aesthetic medicine. If this growth proves anything, it is that there is a huge demand for treatments that keep us young. And it must be said that the results are sometimes spectacular.

But if one thinks about the human body in a holistic way, and wonders what truly changes with these so-called anti-aging treatments, one reaches the conclusion that they are hardly *anti-aging*, because the changes are in appearance only. Spectacular, but superficial. Meanwhile, under the surface, the process of life and aging continues inexorably. That is why some treatments such as Botox or filler injections must be repeated regularly. They improve the appearance but do not eliminate the source of the problem.

This does not mean that aesthetic medical treatments are useless. For many of their users, they may have a positive psychological effect such as improved self-esteem, which is an important part of health and well-being.

However, it is still self-esteem linked to our appearance. How we wish to be seen by others. Conforming to external pressure, to stereotypes placed upon us. Self-esteem that is ultimately based on fulfilling what is expected of us.

But there is a healthier kind of self-esteem and subtler beauty, which is based on accepting ourselves as we are, not placing more importance on appearance than substance, and not giving in to stereotypes and pressures. A self-esteem that comes from inside.

> If we want to change our biological age, and not just the appearance of our chronological age, we will have to alter what happens under the surface, in the depths of our cells.

This dichotomy between external pressure and internal drive is essential when we talk about stopping the aging process. We can settle for appearances, put makeup on our face, and present ourselves to society pretending time does not touch us. But if we want to change our biological age, and not just the appearance of our chronological age, we will have to alter what happens under the surface, in the depths of our cells. We must undertake, like Jules Verne, a journey to the center of our bodies. This is the grand exploration adventure of the 21st century.

How Skin Changes with Age

Epidermis: The outermost layer

△ **Elastin:** Maintains the elasticity of the skin

■ **Dermis:** The deepest layer

○ **Collagen:** Maintains the integrity of the tissue

YOUNG SKIN

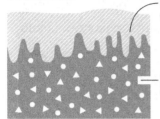

Epidermis and dermis are closely connected

High density of collagen fibers and elastin in the dermis

NATURAL AGING

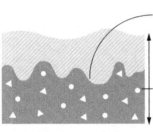

It reduces the amount of fibers that connect the epidermis and the dermis

Fewer collagen fibers and elastin

Skin becomes thinner

PHOTOAGING

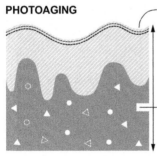

Skin accumulates atypical and inflammatory cells due to the effects of ultraviolet radiation

Collagen fibers and elastin degrade, which accelerates the appearance of wrinkles

Skin becomes thicker

CELLS NEVER SLEEP

THE MICROSCOPIC EFFECTS OF THE PASSAGE OF TIME IN OUR TISSUES

When one begins to consider what happens in the body as we age, the first impression is confusion. If we are guided by common sense, we start with the idea that it is a process of progressive deterioration. But soon, we realize that this idea is too simple. Not everything deteriorates. Or at least not everything deteriorates the same way.

Crystallized intelligence, for example, which is based on knowledge and skills acquired throughout life, improves with experience and therefore with age. The ability to recognize emotions on other people's faces also improves over the years. There are other types of intelligence, however, that do decline.

If we look at what happens in the cells, which are the basic units that form our bodies, the picture that emerges is enormously complex. Dozens of molecules have been identified in the aging process, but it is not clear from the outset what relationship they share.

Are they acting independently, like guerrillas threatening our wellbeing without coordination? Or are we programmed to grow old in a controlled manner—to retire in time to make way for the next generations? The distinction is important, because if they are autonomous guerrillas, it will achieve little to fight just one since others will continue attacking. But if they are organized and there is an alpha molecule in command, we can focus on eliminating it or negotiating with it to stop the aging process.

NOT EVERYTHING DETERIORATES. OR AT LEAST NOT EVERYTHING DETERIORATES THE SAME WAY. CRYSTALLIZED INTELLIGENCE, FOR EXAMPLE, WHICH IS BASED ON KNOWLEDGE AND SKILLS ACQUIRED THROUGHOUT LIFE, IMPROVES WITH EXPERIENCE AND, THEREFORE, WITH AGE. THE ABILITY TO RECOGNIZE EMOTIONS ON OTHER PEOPLE'S FACES ALSO IMPROVES OVER THE YEARS.

Let us begin with telomeres, which we discussed in chapter 1, when we said that there is a test that uses them to calculate biological age. If we can estimate the age of our cells only from the telomeres, it is because they are important. So important, in fact, that the scientists who discovered how they worked received the Nobel Prize in Medicine in 2009.

To explain telomeres, they are often compared to the small plastic cylinders that protect the tip of shoelaces. What telomeres protect are the ends of the chromosomes—in other words, the packets of DNA in the nucleus of our cells. The chromosomes have a shape that resembles an X, with four arms. At the end of each arm of the chromosomes are the protecting telomeres. In the same way the tips on shoelaces become worn out with use, the telomeres wear out each time a cell divides. More precisely, they get shorter.

The longer we have lived, the more times our cells have divided and the shorter our telomeres have become, until they become so short that they can no longer protect the chromosomes. Just as the shoelace frays when the plastic tip wears out, chromosomes fail to function well without telomeres. This has serious consequences for the cells because the chromosomes are essential for their division. So when a cell is left with telomeres that are too short, it stops dividing. It is said to enter a state of *senescence*.

The human body has an antidote to prevent premature shortening of the telomeres. It is an enzyme called telomerase, whose sole function is to repair telomeres. Of course, it does not work with the same dedication for all the cells of the body. In neurons, for example, which are a type of cell that do not divide and, therefore, telomeres do not shorten, it is inactive. In the cells of the wall of the large intestine which divide incessantly, to the point where they renovate every four days, it is always active.

Like anything else that works hard, telomerase is not infallible. Sometimes it behaves in a way it should not, such as in the case of cancerous cells, which can endlessly proliferate thanks to the abundant production of telomerase. And other times, it does not work where it should, as in the cells that enter a state of premature senescence. So even with the telomerase, there is still a progressive shortening of telomeres, the cells enter a state of senescence, and the tissues and organs where these cells are located fall into a decline. This decline is what we perceive as aging.

If all that sounds very technical, have patience. In a few pages, it will all make more sense. To gain a better understanding, we must delve a little further into the fascinating world of cells. That is because telomeres are important factors in the history of aging, but they are not the only ones.

If we look at the part of DNA that is not telomeres, we will see that it accumulates genetic alterations throughout our life. Some of these alterations occur spontaneously because DNA is not a perfectly stable molecule and undergoes small changes unintentionally. Other alterations arise when cells divide and must copy their entire DNA—consisting of approximately three billion letters—so that the two daughter cells have a complete genome each. With so many letters, it is understandable if a typo occurs. In addition, there are the many alterations produced by external aggressions, such as the toxins in tobacco or the ultraviolet rays of the sun. In short, our DNA slowly deteriorates as we live.

Just as we have telomerase to repair the telomeres, our cells have a variety of tools to detect and repair the small breakdowns that occur daily within our DNA. Incidentally, these tools are so important that their discovery led to a Nobel Prize in Chemistry in 2005. But these tools, as happens with telomerase, are not enough to repair all the damage, and with the accumulation of genetic alterations, many of our cells stop working properly because they suffer from a kind of cell disease called genomic instability.

One might think that, because our cells are microscopic, they must be quite simple. Nothing could be further from reality: each of the cells in the body is of astonishing complexity.

One might think that because our cells are microscopic they are simple. Nothing could be further from reality.

There are cells that are complete living beings in themselves. For example, consider bacteria, the most numerous creatures on Earth. Every cell in the body is more complex than bacteria. Each has thousands of proteins that must work in a perfectly coordinated way, like musicians in a symphony orchestra. Each of these proteins must execute the precise note at the right time.

So, beyond the DNA, there are a multitude of molecules in our cells that act in the aging drama. Some are leading actors, while others are more like extras. You have probably heard of free radicals. They have been the villains for years. There is a popular aging theory—called the Theory of Free Radicals, in fact—which accuses them of being the main culprits in the progressive deterioration of health.

At first glance, it is a plausible theory. Free radicals are molecules that cause chemical oxidation reactions in our cells. They are accused of committing serious microscopic crimes, such as oxidative stress, or more broadly, oxidative damage. This damage, which accumulates with age, has been associated with many diseases, such as cancer, atherosclerosis, and Alzheimer's, which has led to the defense of antioxidants as being beneficial to health and the antidote to aging.

But this theory was proposed in the 1950s, when we did not know everything that we know now about the intimate life of our cells. And although the theory has since evolved, investigations conducted in recent years call into question that radicals are bad and antioxidants good.

When an overdose of free radicals was applied to yeast and worms, which are two of the most studied organisms in biology, it was observed, against all odds, that the free radicals lengthened life rather than shortened it. In mice, which are mammals and therefore more similar to us, it is observed that neither do the free radicals accelerate the aging process nor do the antioxidants prolong life. Surprisingly, it has also been observed that smokers are more prone to lung cancer if they take antioxidant supplements than if they do not. All of which suggests that free radicals and oxidation reactions are necessary for the proper functioning of our bodies.

Other molecules, however, seemed to be nice guys until they exposed their dark side. Take the example of the IGF-1 hormone (full name: insulin-like growth factor 1), which is necessary for growth during childhood but accelerates the aging process in adulthood—at least in worms. In fact, the worms with inactive IGF-1 live twice as long, which is the human equivalent of living 150 years in good health.

Another example: the IL-6 protein (or interleukin-6), which is secreted by cells of the immune system and is necessary to combat infections and other beneficial functions. It also seems to favor the aging process.

A group of particularly interesting molecules are the sirtuins, which act as the guardian angels of our cells. We have seven different types of sirtuins, all appearing to be beneficial. The sirtuin 1 (SIRT1), for example, has prolonged life by 44 percent in an experiment conducted with mice. Pharmaceutical companies have begun to develop drugs that mimic its effects, although it is too early to know its applications. Sirtuin 6 (SIRT6) helps repair DNA, among other functions, and has prolonged life by 16 percent in an experiment conducted on mice.

There are many other molecules involved in aging: PGC-1alpha, mTOR, CETP, AMPK, NF-KB...If all these acronyms mean nothing to you, you are not alone. Admittedly, it looks like alphabet soup. The picture that emerges from all this confusion resembles a puzzle. We have many loose pieces on the table, and it is not clear at first glance how they all fit together. What relationship, if any, do DNA lesions have with the different sirtuins? And telomeres with the IGF-1 hormone, or IL-6 protein?

Each of these pieces forms a detail of a larger picture. To understand how it all fits together, we must have a vision of the whole. It is what we will do in the next chapter: begin to put the puzzle together.

Telomeres, the Guardians of the Chromosomes

DNA is organized into chromosomes in the nucleus of the cells

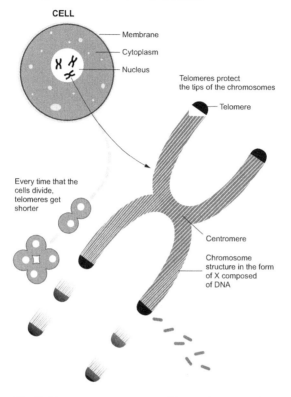

CELL

Membrane

Cytoplasm

Nucleus

Telomeres protect
the tips of the chromosomes

Telomere

Every time that the
cells divide,
telomeres get
shorter

Centromere

Chromosome
structure in the form
of X composed
of DNA

When the telomeres are too
short, the cells lose their ability
to divide

Telomerase is an enzyme that
regenerates the telomeres and
halts their shortening

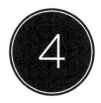

RENEW OR DIE

HOW TISSUE IS BUILT AND MAINTAINED IN THE HUMAN BODY

To have an overall vision, it is useful to remember that we are custodians of genetic material that we have inherited from our parents and that many of us will transmit to our children. These are small links in the long chain of life, which come from a remote past and are heading for a distant future. To transmit from one generation to the next, DNA needs a vessel. DNA takes its time to build this vessel, then it keeps it while it is useful and discards it in the end. This vessel is the body.

Therefore, in human life there is a construction phase, a maintenance phase, and a decline phase. Of course, the human body is capable of much more than simply transmitting DNA. It is capable of feeling, thinking, building cathedrals, and wondering about its place in the universe. Unlike cacti and anacondas, which do not know they are instruments of DNA, we have been given the privilege of enjoying life consciously. Although consciousness, ultimately, has also developed from DNA as another tool to reach the next generation.

In the construction phase, stem cells, which are a type of very particular cells, have a crucial role. They can be compared to a small child, for whom everything is still possible. Perhaps he will become a great farmer, or a soccer player, or an astronaut. Who knows? His entire future is open. Similarly, at the beginning of the life of a stem cell, it can become any of the hundreds of different types of cells we have in the body.

Then, as the child grows, options begin to lessen. We can dismiss the future soccer player, but there is still a wide range of options: doctor, actor, entrepreneur, journalist... Later, the range narrows again. And at the end of the process, there is only one remaining option: the young one will be, let's say, a piano tuner.

The same happens with stem cells as the body takes shape. Initially, they could be any type of cell, then only certain types, then they gradually become more particular, and at the end, they have a single destiny. They will be then, say, liver cells, and proud of it. Not everyone can be a brain cell.

This business of building the body is not solely the DNA's job. Our DNA is the orchestra director. But a director without musicians cannot give life to a symphony. The musicians who interpret the great symphony of life are the proteins and other cell molecules. DNA determines which proteins must act in each moment and in every part of the body. But whether the result is harmonious or chaotic, health or illness, depends on what the proteins do.

There are myriad proteins that work in the construction of the human body. The growth factors—as the name suggests—stimulate growth; the proteins of the Notch family are involved in the development of tissues; the cyclins regulate the division of the cells...There are hundreds of them.

Once the construction of the body is complete, all these musicians—who have played with such spirit and have created a masterpiece—will have to change score and share the stage with the other performers, who have joined for the next piece to begin in the maintenance phase.

In this phase, to ensure good maintenance, two things must happen: replace what does not work, and throw away the garbage. Anyone who has ever had to maintain a house, an orchard, a computer, or a lamp with a burned-out lightbulb knows the deal. One must put in the new bulb and throw away the old. Regenerate and eliminate.

In the human body, the ones in charge of regeneration are the so-called progenitor cells. They are no longer the same stem cells they were at the beginning of life: those that had an open future and could become any type of cell in the body. They are now a more specialized type of cell. Some researchers also call them mother cells because they generate daughter cells. Here, to avoid confusion, we will call them progenitor cells.

They have already chosen what they will do, like the child who became a piano tuner. Once they are committed to being liver progenitor cells, their fate will be to work their entire life, tirelessly, day and night, to regenerate that organ and to keep it working.

This daily regeneration of the progenitor cells occurs in almost all the tissues of the body. Whether it is the skin, the stomach, the kidneys, or the blood, the eliminated cells are replaced by new ones.

This leads to the second requirement. The residue must be removed to keep the house clean. The human body has a sophisticated cleaning brigade in charge of removing and recycling waste.

First, we have the garbage trucks, which in our case are specialized cells called phagocytes that engulf the cells, and cellular debris that must be removed.

They are called phagocytes because they eat *(phage)* cells *(cite)*.

Then the waste must be recycled. We do it through a process called autophagy, which means to eat *(phagy)* its own *(auto)* waste.

We are not explaining all of this because we want to torture you with technical terms, but rather because autophagy plays a central role in the aging process. In fact, recycling waste effectively—meaning, having an efficient autophagy—helps prevent age-related diseases such as osteoarthritis, atherosclerosis, or cancer.

This system of regeneration by the progenitor cells and cleaning through autophagy allows us to maintain good health for most of our life. Its function is to remove cells that have completed their work and must be replaced, in the same way that we must replace worn tires. It also repairs damage caused by external aggressions, such as infections, toxins, or harm caused to our cells by ionizing radiation.

However, there are situations where progenitor cells and autophagy are not enough to repair the damage. If you have ever had surgery, you probably still have a scar. If you look carefully, the scar tissue is not like the skin around it. It does not have the same exact color or texture. This happens because the cells of the scar are not the same as the rest of the skin. They are repair cells, like when we repair a punctured tire with a patch.

This type of repair also happens in internal organs. It is known as fibrosis, because the new tissue that is formed has a fibrous texture. Of course, it does not have the same properties as the original tissue. In the heart, for example, fibrous tissue does not have the contraction capacity of healthy muscle cells. Thus, rather than assisting in pumping out blood, it is a hindrance. In the liver, it cannot fulfill the functions of the original hepatocytes. The same happens in the lungs, pancreas, kidneys...Fibrosis, in essence, is an emergency solution to repair damage, which can later become damage that requires emergency solutions.

With the maintenance and repair systems we have described—progenitor cells, fibrosis, and autophagy—we can live well for decades. If we are part of the Glass Is Half Empty Club and prefer to see the negative side of things, surely we will find reasons to complain: incipient baldness, a tendency to gain weight, unexpected lower back pain. But if we take care of ourselves, the majority of people living in developed economies can enjoy excellent health well into an advanced age.

There will come a point, however, when the body's maintenance and repair mechanisms will begin to fail. Progenitor cells, depleted after having worked so hard for so many years, will lose the ability to regenerate tissues. It will be like retiring. When this occurs, and the progenitor cells can no longer replenish dying cells, they enter a state of senescence. This is not a harmless state. A senescent cell, instead of sitting quietly in a corner of the body, prefers to draw attention. It can no longer create new cells, but it secretes substances that provoke inflammation.

Something similar happens with autophagy. What was originally a cleaning mechanism to keep the body in good condition ends up being overwhelmed and begins to act badly. It is not harmless, either. In fact, all the diseases unique to aging may be initiated or exacerbated by decisions made by our cleaning brigades. Cardiovascular, neurodegenerative diseases, cancers...any of those.

Fibrosis can also be damaging. As we have seen, it creates a type of fibrous tissue that does not replace the role of the original tissue, which can lead to organ failure. But, like the senescence of the progenitor cells and badly regulated autophagy, fibrosis, too, is accompanied by an inflammatory response.

The common element in all these cases is that the mechanisms that should protect us begin to impair us, sometimes with fatal consequences. This is precisely what happens with inflammation. It is a response of the immune system and, therefore, a defense mechanism. But often the cure is worse than the original injury.

Examples of this include when we feel ill due to fever, which is an inflammatory reaction. Or when skin swells and reddens from a mosquito bite, or in more serious cases, when a person gets the flu and suffers a serious complication, which is sometimes even fatal. Or in aging, the declining phase that follows the maintenance phase. In all these cases, inflammation is largely responsible.

This is the point where all the molecules we discussed in earlier chapters, which at first glance looked like random pieces of a puzzle, begin to fit together: free radicals and their antidotes, antioxidants; the telomeres that degrade and the telomerase that rebuilds; sirtuins that prolong the life of mice; interleukins secreted by the immune system; and the IGF-1 that we will discuss in the following chapters.

All of them play a meaningful role in this general life plan with its construction phase and maintenance phase. The maintenance phase is based on regeneration (mother cells), waste management (autophagy), and emergency repairs (fibrosis); in the end, this maintenance system stops functioning well and enters an uncontrolled phase.

If the system works well for decades, why would it not work well for centuries? After all, there are turtles and whales that are over 150 years old. And some trees, which are also living multi-cellular beings, live for over a thousand years. Why not us?

We could say it is because nature stopped caring. We must not lose sight of the fact that nature acts as a company, optimizing resources and maximizing profits. The benefit it seeks is not money; it is the creation of life, and it gave birth to us so we could be its workers. This does not mean that we must accept submissively, but this is the initial role assigned to us in the grand scheme of life on Earth.

In this grand scheme, as we were saying earlier, we are repositories of a small treasure of DNA that we are asked to deliver to the next generation, like athletes in a relay race. It gives us a body to do so and sufficient time to accomplish the mission. During this time, until the end of the reproductive age, we need good health to bequeath our genes to the future.

For us to finish our work, natural selection has provided us with health insurance: the maintenance and repair mechanisms we talked about. But once the reproduction phase is exhausted, we stop being necessary, and our health insurance is not renewed. The maintenance mechanism degrades into a process we call aging.

Of course, human beings can enjoy good health well beyond the childbearing age.

This is true not only in technologically advanced societies, but also among groups of hunter-gatherers living in the Paleolithic period, such as the Hadza of Tanzania or the San of Namibia. They often have children between the ages of twenty and forty-five and can live in very good health well beyond their seventies. Therefore, one might think that we are not programmed to disappear at the end of our reproductive age like other animals.

In reality, humans are peculiar creatures and our phase of reproduction extends beyond the stage of fertility. We have a slower development than other species, and our children require a much longer period of intensive maternal care. Our reproductive strategy is very different from that of lions or penguins, which are moving around by themselves a few weeks after birth and in three or four years can start to reproduce.

Human offspring depend on adult protection for over a decade. They need to be provided with food during the first years of life and, much later, to be taught how to look for it. They need to be educated; they need to be taught how to find water, to recognize dangers, to communicate with each other. There is no other species in the animal kingdom that is as dependent on their parents for so many years as humans are.

NATURE HAS ORGANIZED US INTO EXTENDED FAMILIES AND LARGE SOCIAL GROUPS. IT HAS DONE SO TO PROTECT THE YOUNG, TO HELP THEM REACH ADULTHOOD AND BE ABLE TO HAND THE BATON TO THE NEXT GENERATION. THAT IS WHY WE'VE BEEN GRANTED THE EXCEPTIONAL CLEMENCY TO REACH GRANDPARENTHOOD.

All this cannot be done by the father and mother alone. They need help, as any family in modern urban societies has proven and as our ancestors in the Paleolithic period knew. More so if they are having children every three or four years, as has been the case for most of the history of mankind. And even more so if the father or mother dies prematurely due to a hunting accident or a difficult delivery, as has also been the case.

For this reason, nature has organized us into families and large social groups. It has done so to protect the young, to help them reach adulthood and be able to hand the baton to the next generation. That is why we have been granted the exceptional clemency to reach grandparenthood. Our fertility may decline between forty and fifty years of age, but the reproductive cycle includes three generations and extends to around the age of seventy.

We are not the only ones. Orcas and elephants also live

in large social groups, formed by animals of three or four generations, guided by older females that stand out for their crystallized intelligence (the type of intelligence that increases with age, if you remember from chapter 1). What they have in common with us is that their young take more than a decade to reach reproductive age and are very dependent on their mother and adult members of the herd in their first years of life. This confirms that it is this need to protect, feed, and educate the young that allows—or rather forces—individual species to have grandparents.

If any lesson can be learned from all this, it is how important grandparents are to human beings. Without grandparents, there would be no humanity. In a time where we value elders so little, it is a lesson worth remembering.

Mother Cells Build and Regenerate the Human Body

1. In the moment of fertilization, the union of egg and sperm form the zygote

The zygote is the mother of all the cells that the human body has throughout life

2. The embryo develops from the zygote. For the first few days, your cells have the ability to become any cell in the body

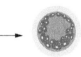

3. As the embryo develops, the cells begin to specialize. Mother cells can generate some types of cells but not others

4. In an adult, mother cells are specialized. At this point, they are called progenitor cells. Most can only create a specific type of cell, which allows the tissues to regenerate throughout life

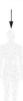

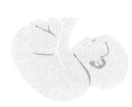

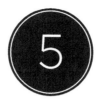

THE ARROW OF TIME

AGING CANNOT BE REVERSED, BUT IT CAN BE STOPPED

We said in the previous chapter that we do not want to torture you with technical terms. Well, in this chapter we are going to introduce another term: homeostasis.

It is what makes a biological system like our bodies remain in a state of internal balance that enables it to function and have stability. The word comes from *homeo* (similar) and *stasis* (balance). This concept is essential to understanding both our health (which depends on a good homeostasis) and the aging process (which is the degradation of our homeostasis systems).

To facilitate understanding, we will give you some examples. A classic example is body temperature, which in our case has its point of balance at 36.5 degrees Celsius (97.7 degrees Fahrenheit). If it goes up, the body is responsible for lowering it. It if goes down, the body is responsible for raising it. We have a highly sophisticated system of regulation that includes temperature sensors distributed throughout the body (for example, in the skin), a control center in the brain (specifically, in the hypothalamus), and corrective mechanisms (such as shivering or seeking the sun to raise the temperature, and sweating and seeking the shade to lower it). In older people, the system of temperature perception degrades, and it is common for older people to be cold in situations when young people are hot.

Another illustrative example is blood pressure, which is complexly regulated by the heart, the kidneys, the brain, and the blood vessels. Or the amount of water in the blood, which is regulated by the feeling of thirst which leads us to drink, and urine to evacuate the excess. Or sleep regulation, which keeps us awake when we have slept enough, but makes us sleep again when go into deficit.

Hunger, sleep, cold, heat, thirst, or fatigue...All are reactions of adaptation to maintain our internal balance, or homeostasis. As in Lampedusa's *The Leopard*: whatever changes, everything must remain the same.

When the protagonist in Oscar Wilde's novel *The Portrait of Dorian Gray* sells his soul for eternal youth, he desires a whole-body homeostasis. He is not unlike actors and many other people who use medical treatments to maintain their bodies without the appearance of change. The goal is to stay the same and to remain just as healthy and attractive as in their youth.

However, this is not possible, nor will it ever be. Biology does not allow it, nor does physics.

In biology, homeostasis requires a constant state of initial balance and three elements to maintain it. It must have sensors, a control center, and corrective mechanisms to restore the state of balance. This is what happens with temperature, the level of sugar in the blood, or the amount of fat in our bodies. That is why it is hard to lose weight and not regain it. The body tends to return to the starting point before the weight loss, and we must find strategies to deceive the system of weight homeostasis and establish a new balance.

But this is not what happens with age. First, there is no point of initial balance. At what point should we set the age? Maybe around twenty years old, at the end of the developmental stage, when other balance points such as weight and organ size are set? Why not a little later, let's say around thirty years of age, when we have accumulated enough experience to help our children get ahead? Ah, but we forget that humans need grandparents to help with the upbringing. Perhaps we should establish the point of balance for later? Around fifty years old?

Any of these scenarios would lead us to a situation where a new human being is born while older ones remain. But just as in the skin or kidneys or any organ, cells are replaced by new ones when they have completed their mission. In every ecosystem, living beings must die to make way for those being born. This is how nature works.

There is a type of cell that refuses to die: cancer cells, which have developed schemes to try to achieve immortality. But all they manage to do is damage the ecosystem, which is the body in which they were born. Similarly, any species which finds something like immortality will destroy the ecosystem that it lives in and threaten its very survival. This directly affects human beings: do we want to maintain this biosphere in balance, or would we rather act like cancer cells? The answer to this question, or lack thereof, influences the wellbeing of people who will live in the future and will judge without indulgence the excesses of our generation.

Returning to the topic of health, the fact is that we do not have evolution on our side if we wish to establish an age after which we no longer change, like the temperature set at 36.5 degrees Celsius. What we would be asking is to detain evolution. Stop time.

This leaves us in the hands of physics, which oversees time. The truth is that no one has managed to satisfactorily explain why time flows from the past into the future but cannot do so in reverse. But there is something that, to a lesser extent, is well known. It is the second law of thermodynamics.

This law does not allow for what has become disorganized to become reorganized and be the same as it was before. To be precise, it does not allow it in a closed system without external energy input. If the system is simple—for example, a shuffled deck of cards—we can put them in order if we apply a bit of energy and have a little patience. But if the system is complex, as are the living beings that interact in ecosystems, there is no turning back. The organization of the system becomes irrecoverable.

That is why the egg that falls to the ground cannot be put back together and the elephant shot by a bullet does not rise again. There is no return from death; the second law does not allow it. Neither is an extinct species born again nor an ecosystem that is destroyed formed again. This is why it does not make sense to clone mammoths or dinosaurs. The ecosystem on which they depended cannot be recreated. And in the human body, which is a small ecosystem, the changes that accumulate with age are irreversible.

THERE IS NO RETURN FROM DEATH...NEITHER IS AN
EXTINCT SPECIES BORN AGAIN NOR AN ECOSYSTEM
THAT IS DESTROYED FORMED AGAIN. THIS IS
WHY IT MAKES NO SENSE TO CLONE MAMMOTHS
OR DINOSAURS. THE ECOSYSTEMS ON WHICH
THEY DEPENDED CANNOT BE RECREATED.

We say it unanimously. This distinction is important. Because there are partial changes that are reversible. The eye operated on for a cataract in which a new lens is implanted, the tooth with a repaired cavity, the parts of the epidermis where wrinkles are eliminated...these are all examples of reversible damage. But while these problems are being corrected, life continues its course and other damages accumulate.

The aging process is what doctors call a multi-factorial process, which means that it is not the result of a single cause, but a sum of different causes. Even if one of the causes is eliminated, the others will continue to act.

Think about the difference between infections and cardiovascular diseases. An infection has a single cause: for example, a virus or bacteria. If it is successfully treated with an antibiotic or antiviral, and with the help of our immune system, the infection disappears. Problem solved.

This does not mean it is easy—there are infections resistant to treatment—but it is doable.

Cardiovascular diseases are different. There are thousands of molecules that regulate the activity of the heart, the blood composition, and the functioning of arteries and veins. These thousands of molecules work in a coordinated manner, without one commanding the others. We know the role of cholesterol is very important, but so are those of insulin, calcium, coagulation factors, the TGF-beta...There are myriad molecules involved. Even if two or three slow down, the others will continue pushing.

Aging progresses similarly. It is also multi-factorial. But instead of being limited to the circulatory system, it extends to the whole body. So it is even more difficult to address.

Where does all this leave us when it comes to birthdays and maintaining full physical and mental shape, as we promised you on the cover of the book?

An ideal anti-aging treatment could aspire to keep us unchanging, like Dorian Gray in Oscar Wilde's novel. But we have already seen this is not possible. It is a strategy doomed to failure and frustration because life is movement, a process of permanent change. Detaining this change would mean stopping life itself.

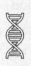

DNA
Contains the genetic instructions to build and operate the human body

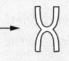

- Shortening of telomeres
- Epigenetic alterations
- Genome instability

Proteins
Molecules that build with genetic instructions from DNA

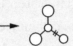

- Defective proteins

Metabolism
Stands for the chemical reactions produced between molecules in the body

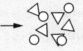

- Oxidative stress

Organism
The observable traits and characteristics of a living being are called phenotype

Aging: What we perceive in the human body as a result of processes that occur on a microscopic scale

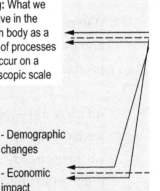

Society
Interpersonal relationships are key to people's health

- Demographic changes

- Economic impact

Major health challenges, such as aging, can only be addressed successfully when they take place at all levels of biological organization, from the DNA to the whole of society

Genomic

- Cellular senescence
- Exhaustion of progenitor cells

Proteomics

- Less autophagy
- More inflammation

Metabolomics

Medical Specialties

Social Sciences

If we cannot stay the same, we could aspire to rejuvenate. Go back in time. Although it is not possible for the entire body, we have seen that it is possible for specific organs. The lens, the tooth, the epidermis...Why not the liver, the heart, the brain? With effective rejuvenating treatment for enough organs, and for sufficiently important organs, we could achieve a large-scale effect for the whole body. In fact, this is the goal of regenerative medicine, a field of research that studies the regeneration of damaged organs through stem cells and bioengineering techniques. But even if these investigations are successful and the hope for stem cells is fulfilled, the second law will ultimately impose itself. As far as we know, nothing in the history of the universe has escaped this law.

If we cannot stop or go back, there is only one other option: to move slowly. Slow down the aging process. This, as we shall see in the next chapters, is possible. Throughout the history of mankind, the aging process has always been seen as inevitable, something against which nothing could be done except to resign ourselves. Now, for the first time, we are beginning to have prevention strategies to delay it.

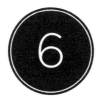

EXPIRATION DATE

THE MICROSCOPIC EFFECTS OF THE PASSAGE OF TIME IN OUR ORGANS

To win a battle, it is always better to know who you are facing. Know your enemy, as Green Day sang. If we want to stop the aging process, it is useful to pause for a moment to clarify how it progresses. This is done by observing what happens in the privacy of our cells, not only at the microscopic level, as we have done in chapters 3 and 4, but also at the macroscopic level, examining what happens to large organs and the body as a whole.

To some of you, this may seem like a no-brainer. At some point, we have all experienced what it feels like to become older. We note changes in our physical appearance, our vitality, and our enthusiasm in doing things. Physical effort is more difficult. There comes a day where we can no longer do somersaults or handstands. The capacity for surprise atrophies and resignation develops, because it is a process both physical and psychological. But beyond these vague ideas, it is interesting how little we know about how the body changes with age.

The American Nathan Shock (1906–1989) was the first to realize how ignorant we are about aging. Or at least the first to study the issue scientifically. He was a pioneer recognized as one of the fathers of gerontology, i.e., the scientific study of old age. If not for Shock, you might not be reading this book today, because we would not know enough to write it.

Shock had the great idea of investigating aging in a longitudinal study, which means analyzing how people evolve over time. This is not easy or low-cost. It requires convincing participants in the study to collaborate for years and an organization to keep in touch with them, and finding someone to pay for the whole setup—which in his case was something of questionable usefulness that no one had tried before. It would have been much easier and more affordable to do a cross-sectional study: i.e., analyze a large group of people of different ages all at once. But then he would not have found out everything he discovered.

Shock began the Baltimore Longitudinal Study of Aging in 1958. He started with 260 volunteers that, at the time of enrollment, were between twenty and ninety-six years old. In the following years and decades, the study expanded to hundreds of volunteers, who allowed him to conduct exhaustive tests every two years. They agreed to let him to observe everything—from their muscle strength to their aerobic capacity, from their walking pace to their mental agility, from their bone density to their skeletal shape, as well as their vision, hearing, cholesterol, weight, height, blood pressure, mood...Men allowed their prostate and testosterone to be examined, and women, their estrogen levels. They allowed everything to be looked at and questioned. If they smoked, drank, ate, how much they slept... The best compliment to the Baltimore study is that when Nathan Shock died, his project continued. It continues today under the auspices of the National Institute on Aging, a division of the U.S. National Institutes of Health.

Shock demonstrated that aging and disease are different processes. While it is true that the risk of disease increases with age, there are people that age without becoming ill. Therefore, healthy aging is not a utopia. It is not just a positive expression that we say to delude ourselves. It is a goal to which many can aspire.

The study also showed how every person and every organ ages differently. There is no normal aging pace. There is no predefined schedule to which we are bound. If you believe that you can read the future in the palm of your hand, in the lines of health and life, stop lying to yourself. Science says otherwise: the future is not written. We have a draft of the future in our DNA, but we change it every day with the decisions we make, with our successes and with our mistakes.

Even so, there are some general patterns that we can't escape, such as the speed at which we walk. Studies such as Baltimore have found that gait slows down with age and is one of the indicators that more reliably predict the risk of death in subsequent years. This has been observed not only in elderly people, where the risk of death is predictably higher when they have more trouble walking, but it has also been observed in adults who appear to be healthy.

The strength in our hands also declines with age. Both in men and in women, the more strength we have, the more likely we are to enjoy good health in the years to come. In the first major study on the subject, more than 6,000 people in Hawaii between the ages of forty-five and sixty-eight underwent a manual test of strength in the framework of cardiovascular health research. It was a longitudinal study, like Baltimore. Twenty-five years later, those who had shown more strength in the test had better health and were more autonomous: more likely to go shopping and carry more than four kilos (nine pounds), do physical work like cleaning the garden or the garage, go up and down stairs, or walk at a good pace.

WHILE IT IS TRUE THAT THE RISK OF DISEASE INCREASES WITH AGE, THERE ARE PEOPLE THAT AGE WITHOUT BECOMING ILL. THEREFORE, HEALTHY AGING IS NOT A UTOPIA. IT'S A GOAL THAT MANY CAN ASPIRE TO ACHIEVE.

At first glance, it is surprising. How is it possible that by examining the strength of our grip with a simple test that lasts only a few seconds, we can predict what will happen to us twenty-five years later? Remember the palm reading we mentioned before and said had no scientific basis? The prediction of health based on the strength of our grip, however, does have a foundation. Multiple studies have confirmed that there is a correlation between strength and health. The most comprehensive and definitive study analyzed nearly 140,000 individuals from seventeen countries who were between the ages of thirty-five and seventy at the beginning of the study. The results show that, not only in older people but also in middle-aged adults, the stronger the grip, the lower the risk of death in the next four years. In fact, manual force predicts the risk of cardiovascular disease even more accurately than blood pressure.

The explanation lies in the muscles. There will come a point when we reach an advanced age that our strength will fail us. We do not know when it will happen, because that varies for each person. But we know that, unless we have an accident or premature illness, that day will come. When this happens, it will be harder to walk, prepare food, get dressed, and even breathe. Everything will be harder. We will lose autonomy and require help. And our strength will fail us sooner or later based on the health and strength of our muscles.

To a middle-aged person, this doesn't seem like a big issue, since they tend to have more than enough strength to do their daily activities.

But when you are asked to squeeze a dynamometer to measure your grip strength, it can be assessed whether you have a wide margin of safety or just enough strength.

This margin of safety is like a strength reserve: a reserve that will be consumed as the years go by. It is like checking how much gas is left in the car halfway through a trip. We can drive around with a quarter of a tank, but we know the gas will run out faster than if we had half a tank.

With a vehicle, all we must do is refuel, but it's not as easy with the human body. Having an active life, in which the muscles must work every day in the same way organs such as the heart, liver, or kidneys work toward the common good, is one way to avoid using up the reserve too fast. Long-term health insurance.

This does not mean that we must run to join a gym and start doing sets worthy of bodybuilders. Going to the gym is highly recommended if you like, but it is not the only way to keep a good reserve of strength. Too much muscle also poses risk. There are cases of injury. They are few, but they are there, such as the acquired muscle becoming so strong that it hurts itself because it tears from the tendon to the bone.

This means that, for creating a reserve of strength in middle-aged people, a sedentary lifestyle is counterproductive long term because it cuts our day-to-day safety margin for overcoming potential health problems in the future.

And it is a reminder of how important it is to maintain muscle health. Muscles have been vilified for years as second players in the human body, as if they were instruments of force and nothing more. If the brain is the headquarters of intelligence, the muscles are the force. Ergo, the muscles must be dumb. In recent years, we have discovered that this view is incorrect. Muscles are sophisticated tissues that, when exercised, secrete beneficial molecules to the whole body.

> Muscles are sophisticated tissues that, when exercised, secrete beneficial molecules to the whole body.

The progressive depletion of muscular reserve also explains the decline of speed as age progresses. People may not walk faster because they think they do not need to. Step by step, without hurry but without pause, we can get everywhere. But if we do not walk faster because we cannot, then eventually we will go more slowly because the reserves are depleting.

In fact, the muscle mass in the human body tends to remain stable between the third and fifth decade of life and then goes into decline, as found in the Baltimore study. The muscles are not the only ones that tend to atrophy. Organs such as kidneys, lungs, the brain, and the heart also lose mass and, little by little, spend their reserve.

When analyzing the oxygen consumption of the body by age, we note that it goes into decline around forty-five years of age, coinciding with the reduction of muscle mass. Forty-five is an average. As stated above, the chronological age does not correspond with the biological, and the decline doesn't affect everyone at the same time. Whether it is before forty-five or after, the phenomenon is the same: the less oxygen the muscles need, the less that the lungs and blood transport. Therefore, there is a synchronized decline in the performance of the muscles, lungs, and heart, confirming once again that in the human body, everything is connected.

And because everything is connected, there is no system in

the body that escapes this coordinated decline of functions. Think about the immune system and its ability to combat infections, eliminate tumor cells, or heal wounds—all medical issues to which older people are more vulnerable. In the nervous system, quick reaction and learning capacity are impacted. In the endocrine system, the production of multiple hormones suffers, as in the drastic example of estrogen in women and gradual drop of testosterone in men. In the musculoskeletal system, we see the loss of bone density and muscle mass, which makes us more vulnerable to injuries. Even without injuries, our joints tend to lose flexibility; the intervertebral discs that act as shock absorbers between the vertebrae lose fluid and become thinner; the arches of the feet tend to become flatter.

All these changes affect our body shape and our movements. That is why people lose height as they get older, at a rate of an inch per decade beginning at age forty. The arms and legs become thinner due to the loss of muscle mass, while our trunk tends to increase in diameter. The loss of muscle mass and bone density and fat redistribution imply that, as a rule, men begin to lose weight around the age of fifty-five while women begin to lose weight at the age of sixty-five, though those details vary largely from person to person.

Along with the changes in body shape, with age our movements also become slower and more unstable. We lose our sense of balance and have a greater tendency to stumble. If you want to prove this, take this simple test: stand up and try balancing yourself on one leg for thirty seconds. You can choose the leg that is most comfortable for you. The only rule is that only one foot may be in contact with the ground. Is it easy? Okay, now close your eyes and repeat the test. Not so easy anymore, right? If you can, ask someone to time how long you can stand like that.

Typically, a person between thirty and forty years of age can hold themselves for about twenty seconds with their eyes closed. Between the ages of forty to fifty, they probably won't be able to last longer than twelve. A decade more, and this will go down to eight seconds. Another ten years, between the ages of sixty and seventy, and they will fall at five seconds. Balance is proven to be an ability that deteriorates with age.

This may seem surprising. Balance depends very little on physical force, so the weakening of muscles should not harm our sense of balance. And it doesn't. What happens is that balance is controlled by the vestibular apparatus in the interior of the ears, which also breaks down with age. The vestibular apparatus is connected to regions of the brain that allow us to react and recover our balance if we're falling, but the brain also loses capacity for reaction and coordination over the years, which does not help us regain balance when stumbling. Our sense of balance also helps our vision by indicating to the brain what the spatial position of the body is. That's why maintaining balance with our eyes closed is more difficult than with our eyes open. But our vision also deteriorates as we get older. To sum it up, the older we get, the less balance we have.

That may seem like nothing but bad news. Surely you are not surprised. Anyone who has seen his or her parents or grandparents age has been witness to this process. The loss of strength, the slowing down, the unsteady walking...

> We can alter the pace at which we age. We can stop it or, depending on what we do, even accelerate it.

And, truly, it is not such bad news. If you stop and think about it, it is actually pretty good. Because, if anything was proven by the Baltimore study and all the longitudinal studies conducted on the aging process, it is that we all age differently, each of us at our own pace. And that this rate depends largely on what we do when we find ourselves well and in full form, on what we do decades before we start to decay, on our actions and our decisions at fifty, forty, thirty years old, or even before. This is the good news. We can alter the pace at which we age. We can stop it or, depending on what we do, even accelerate it. In the next chapters, we will see how we can change it.

The body atrophies with age...

 Men

Age (years) 50   60   70   80

Average height (cm)

Diameter of the forearm (mm)

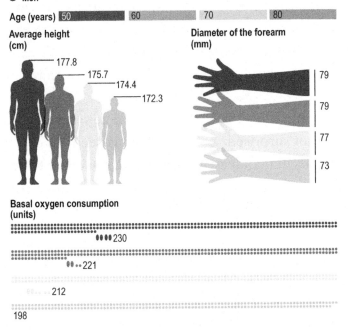

177.8
175.7
174.4
172.3

79
79
77
73

Basal oxygen consumption (units)

230
221
212
198

...but staying in shape delays the decline

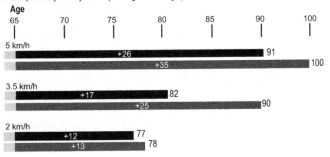 Men ♀ Women

Life expectancy at 65 years depending on walking speed

Age							
65	70	75	80	85	90	100	

5 km/h
+26   91
+35   100

3.5 km/h
+17   82
+25   90

2 km/h
+12   77
+13   78

Source: Baltimore Longitudinal Study of Aging (US data) and JAMA (US data).

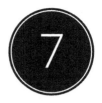

SECRETS OF THE CENTENARIANS

GENETICS DETERMINE HOW WE LIVE

You may have heard of Jeanne Calment. She is an extraordinary woman. What is most extraordinary is that she led a perfectly ordinary life and still lived to be 122 years old. That is 122 years, five months, and fourteen days to be exact, or a total of 44,724 days. It is a Guinness World record. She is the person who, until now, has had the longest life. If someone somewhere has lived longer, it is not documented. How did she manage it?

Like so many people in her time, Jeanne Calment smoked. She smoked from the ages of 21 to 117—almost a century of tobacco—which also makes her the person in the world to have smoked the longest. This is another Guinness record.

Though she rode a bike until the age of 100, she was not particularly worried about her health or being in shape. She would eat, she said, about a kilo (2.20 lb.) of chocolate a week. She also liked port wine and seasoned her food abundantly with olive oil. However, she was a very quiet woman. She would joke, for she certainly had a sense of humor, about why her name was Calment: because she was calm. She would also say, in yet another example of her sense of humor, "I have ever only had one wrinkle, and I'm sitting on it." Clearly, quite a character.

Jeanne Calment was born in Arles, in the south of France, in 1875. During that time, it was common to die young of tuberculosis or pneumonia or complications during childbirth, before antibiotics and modern hygiene. At the time, there were so many deadly infections and unexpected trauma, so many emergencies and sudden deaths, and prevention was unheard of. This was a time when there were no phones, or cars on the streets, the first airplane had not flown, and the Eiffel Tower had not yet been built. Nearly prehistoric times.

She met Van Gogh when the painter first moved to the city. She even sold him some coloring pencils when she was around twelve or thirteen years old and Van Gogh came into her father's shop. Looking at pictures of her youth, it is surprising how she always seemed young for her age. When she was twenty years old, she could have passed for a fifteen-year-old girl, and at forty, for a woman of twenty-five. When she was ninety, she looked like she wasn't a day over eighty.

Calment was a widow with no heirs. She had lost her only child to pneumonia and her only grandson to a car accident. She closed a deal with lawyer André François Raffray, a man around the same age as her grandson. Raffray, who was forty-seven years old, agreed to pay 2,500 francs a month for the rest of Calment's life, in exchange for keeping her apartment when she died. This was a bad deal for the lawyer, who ended up paying more than what the apartment was worth to begin with. What made it such a bad deal was that he was never able to enjoy it: when he died at seventy-seven, Jeanne Calment was still alive. She enjoyed good health until the age of 114, when she broke her femur during a fall and they had to operate, probably making her the oldest person to ever go through surgery. She was lucid in her last days, although at the end of her life she was practically blind and deaf and could barely communicate.

A case such as that of Jeanne Calment does invite us to wonder why some people can get to such advanced ages without apparent effort and others cannot. Is there something special in the functioning of the body that allows them to escape the ills that normally punish the rest of humanity? Were they luckier in the genetic lottery draw that occurs every time an egg and a sperm shuffle their genes? Or is there something more? Is there something that is not only hereditary, but is related to lifestyle, or maybe diet, or the quality of air we breathe, or the immune system, or our resistance to stress? Anything that might give the rest of humanity a clue as to what we can do to live longer and better?

There are not many centenarians: about one person in every six thousand, according to data from the United States. Or, 170 of every million people, if you are better with large numbers. There are not many, but there are enough to study and draw some conclusions.

In recent years, as interest in understanding how we age has increased, studies of centenarians have started in different regions of the world. Examples include the Japanese island of Okinawa, which is one of the areas with a higher life expectancy; Sydney, Australia, where the number of centenarians in 2020 is expected to exceed 12,000, making them the age group that is increasing in population the fastest; and Spain, where the genome of centenarians has been analyzed to try to understand what is so special about them.

Out of all the studies, the most complete is the New England Centenarian Study in the United States, which began in 1994 with forty-six people from the Boston area to investigate Alzheimer's disease, and has since expanded to more than 2,500 people from across the United States to study all aspects of aging.

The first observation that emerges from these studies is that extreme longevity is grouped by families. A person is more likely to become a centenarian if the father or mother, or any of the grandparents or siblings, also lived to be over one hundred years old. In the case of Jeanne Calment, her father lived to be ninety-three and her mother eighty-six, which were exceptional ages for a time of such poor sanitary conditions and where medicine was based more on faith than science.

According to the data from the New England study, if a man has a brother who has lived more than a hundred years, his possibilities to be a centenarian are seventeen times higher than other men of his generation. Similar results have been observed in other studies of extreme longevity in Denmark, Australia, and Japan. If the propensity to live many years is hereditary, this means that there must be genes that influence longevity.

That is no surprise. Just stop and think for a moment how longevity works in the animal kingdom and it is easy to realize that dogs can live up to fifteen years; cats, twenty years; macaws for over seventy years; Galapagos turtles for more than 150 years. They may live less if they get an infection or an attack or some other animal eats them. However, even if nothing happens that may cause a premature death, there is a limit to how long an animal can live. This limit depends on each species. It is decided from the moment one is born cat, turtle, macaw, or human. It is like a maximum potential life that can be reduced but cannot be increased. It is written in the genome of each species and does not depend on the cat's quality of life, but on the fact that it is a cat. This limit must be in the genes.

But when researchers searched for the genes that regulate longevity, they proved to be more difficult to identify than expected. To search for them requires the most advanced techniques of genome analysis, which allow the sequencing of a person's entire DNA and comparison of it with that of others. The complete genome of centenarians has been compared with that of people of average longevity in the hope of finding the genes responsible for the difference. With 3 billion pieces of DNA in the human genome and more than 20,000 genes, it has been a bit like looking for a needle in a haystack. And the needle has yet to appear.

What we have learned is that there is no single gene that has a great influence on longevity, but there are many of little influence.

Still, the search has not been in vain. This is how science works. When things do not go as expected, that's when we tend to learn the most. What we have learned is that there is no single gene that has a great influence on longevity, but that there are many that have a small influence. According to the results of the New England study, there are at least 130 genes that influence how we live. These are 130 genes, possibly more, in which we have found significant differences between centenarians and the rest of the population. None of them alone guarantee a long life. It is the sum of many small actions of many different genes, which allows the adding of years and years of good health.

It is worth wondering what these genes do. Perhaps we can develop treatments that mimic their effects. Or maybe we can alter our lifestyle in a way that develops their activity. Or in the future, we can edit our DNA cells to prolong life.

One of the first ones to be identified, and which has a more significant influence on longevity, is the APOE gene. The full name, if you like the tongue twister or want to do a little exercise of memory to keep your brain in shape, is apolipoprotein E. Like any other gene, it is responsible for the production of a protein. In this case, this protein is essential to the management of cholesterol and fats in the human body. Interestingly, we do not all have the same APOE protein. There are three main forms of the protein in the population. It is like having three different car models. All are good, but not all are equally good.

Depending on the model we get in the genetic lottery, we have either a greater or lower risk of suffering Alzheimer's disease. We also have a higher or lower risk of cardiovascular diseases. Alzheimer's and cardiovascular diseases are an interesting coincidence, because they are precisely two processes associated with aging. And it just so happens that both are associated with a protein that regulates cholesterol and fat.

But APOE, as we were saying, is just one of the many genes that influence how we live. What do the others do? Among centenarians of Okinawa, Germany, and Hawaii, it has been found that another gene also intervenes. It's called FOXO3 and is related to insulin activity and, therefore, the management of the sugar in the body. It is also related to the elimination of free radicals, which are molecules that accumulate with aging. But it does not seem to have anything to do with cholesterol and APOE. This confirms that longevity is a complex trait that does not depend on a single switch, but is regulated by various processes without an apparent connection between them.

An important detail is that the longer a person's life is, the more his or her genetic inheritance influences its longevity. When genetic traits that increase the risk of disease associated with age, such as cardiovascular disease, cancer, or Alzheimer's, are analyzed, it has been observed that these traits also affect centenarians, just like the rest of the population. But centenarians have been graced with more genetic traits that protect them. This allows them to reach advanced ages in good health, watching others of their generation suffer from the diseases from which they have been spared.

IF SOMEONE THINKS THAT IT IS NOT WORTH LIVING MANY YEARS BECAUSE THAT SIMPLY MEANS LIVING LONGER WITH POOR HEALTH, THEY ARE WRONG. THE NONAGENARIANS, CENTENARIANS, AND SUPERCENTENARIANS DEMONSTRATE EXACTLY THE OPPOSITE: THE LONGER WE LIVE, THE LESS TIME WE SPEND SICK.

We may have all heard someone say something like, "My grandfather smoked his entire life, ate eggs with bacon every day, and still lived to be ninety-five years old!" Followed by the quip, "So maybe tobacco and eggs and bacon aren't that bad after all." Well, congratulations about grandfather, but that conclusion is incorrect. It is not that tobacco and excesses in diet are not dangerous, it is just that this grandfather had the luck of being super-protected from the aggressions that punish most of the population. Like Jeanne Calment, who could smoke up until the age of 117 without being affected.

It is precisely this protective effect that is even stronger among supercentenarians, the people who live to be over 110 years old. It is estimated that only one of every thousand centenarians will get to be a supercentenarian. There are very few. But they have an important lesson to teach us.

According to the New England study, which has collected samples from more than one hundred supercentenarians, they are only affected by diseases associated with aging during the last five years of their life. They are, therefore, on average, perfectly healthy beyond the age of 105.

In nonagenarians in the United States, the average time spent with diseases associated with age is 9 percent of their life, almost ten years. And in the whole of the population, also in the United States, it amounts to 18 percent, about fifteen years.

Therefore, if someone thinks that it is not worth it to live a long life because that simply means living longer with poor health, they are wrong. The nonagenarians, centenarians, and supercentenarians demonstrate exactly the opposite: the longer we live, the less time we spend being sick.

Extreme Longevity is Accessible to Few

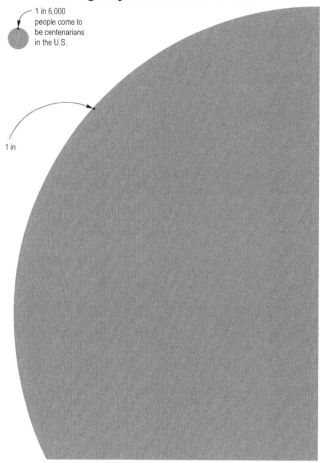

1 in 6,000 people come to be centenarians in the U.S.

1 in

The Longer We Live, the Fewer Years Spent in Poor Health

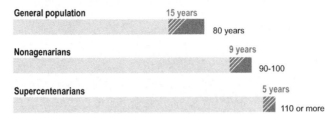

Years lived with poor health

General population — 15 years — 80 years

Nonagenarians — 9 years — 90-100

Supercentenarians — 5 years — 110 or more

Probability of Centenarians Getting a Disease Vs. the General Population

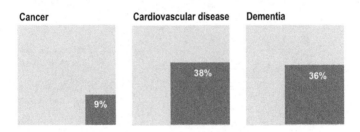

Cancer — 9%

Cardiovascular disease — 38%

Dementia — 36%

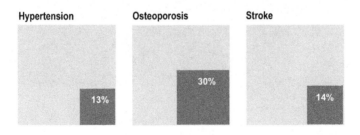

Hypertension — 13%

Osteoporosis — 30%

Stroke — 14%

Source: New England Centenarian Study

THE BLUE ZONES

HOW ENVIRONMENT AFFECTS OUR LONGEVITY

If one could choose where one is born, many would ask for a place with blue skies and mild climate, where nature is generous and gives us varied and tasty foods, where society is fair and cares about educating our children well and taking good care of our elders, and where everyone helps the community to the best of their ability and the community accepts them just as they are. This is a place where people live in peace, with respect and without stress. We're not talking about an imaginary Eden. These places exist. And they are, not coincidentally, some of the places where the highest life expectancy in the world is recorded.

One does not choose the place where one is born, just like we do not choose the parents we have. We get what we get, and we adapt the best we can. Parents give us our genetic inheritance. Our place of origin gives us the environment in which we grow. Genes and environment are the two major variables that regulate human life.

For decades, they have been considered unrelated variables. In scientific literature, we find phrases such as "intelligence is 58 percent genetic and 42 percent environmental." The same has been said of the tendency for obesity, the risk of heart failure, and even sexual orientation. It was published that genes on the X chromosome are linked to male homosexuality. This theory was found to be overly simplistic. In the twentieth century, before the age of the genome, any trait was susceptible to being divided into a ratio of genetic and environmental percentages. This gives us an idea of how ignorant we were fifteen years ago.

It's not that we know everything now. But at least we learned that genetics and environment are intertwined. No man is an island, as the poet John Donne wrote. We all live in an environment that changes us. We get a genetic inheritance with instructions to build and operate our bodies.

This genetic heritage defines what we can become: our maximum potential, maximum longevity, or maximum height, or strength, or creativity...Whatever you like. But then, the environment regulates the functioning of the genes in our cells. Depending on the environment, the genes we have received will either work or not. They will either be activated or silenced. We will either discover our full potential or only get halfway there.

> Genes depend on the environment to function or not, to be activated or silenced, and to determine whether we develop our full potential or stay stunted.

When we talk about environment, we tend to think about the external factors that affect our entire body, either for good or bad. That is, the air we breathe, the food we eat, the stress caused by a bad boss or always rushing everywhere. All this plays an important role in how our DNA works.

But the effects of the environment occur at a microscopic scale in the privacy of the cells. Have you ever wondered why a liver cell is different from a heart cell if they have the same genome? This is because each cell's environment in the human body is different. The molecules and the forces to which the cells are exposed guide them in their development to activate certain genes and silence others. It is almost as if they are educating the cells. Just like some people train to be doctors and others journalists, some cells are formed to work in the heart and others to work in the liver.

It is possible that the doctor could have been a journalist and the journalist a doctor had they chosen different paths when young. The same holds true for cells. Both are equipped with the same DNA and could have been whatever they wanted, but once they have committed to a career in the liver or the heart, there is no turning back.

All this, as you can imagine, has its own jargon among biologists. It is said that the DNA has an epigenetic regulation. This is a word that seems to be here to stay, like other words that our great-grandparents did not know: *genome, laser,* or *internet.* Epigenetic regulation refers to that which acts on (*epi* in Greek) the genes. In fact, it is located literally on top of them. They are molecules that attach themselves to the DNA, with a Judo-like grip, to block the genes that must remain inactive.

That is the end of the theory. You might wonder how this relates to aging and longevity. The answer can be found on the island of Sardinia, Italy. You may have been there. With a privileged position in the middle of the Mediterranean, pleasant climate almost year-round, white sands, clear waters, and beautiful beaches, Sardinia has become a popular tourist destination in recent decades. The answer lies not in the tourist areas or those nearest to the sea, but in the steep mountains at the center of the island.

Belgian demographer Michel Poulain and Italian biomedical researcher Gianni Pes identified a population in Sardinia with an exceptionally high proportion of centenarians. They were located in the Barbagia region. Poulain and Pes took a map, drew a border around the delimited areas, and traced it with blue ink, causing the mountains and valleys where those people lived to become known as *the blue zone.* Their demographic study, conducted in 2000, revealed that 1 out of 196 people born in the blue zone of Sardinia between 1880 and 1900 was a centenarian, making it then the place with the highest proportion of centenarians in the world.

Two years later, the American explorer Dan Buettner embarked on a project to find other places with exceptional longevity rates. He got funding from the National Geographic Society and the National Institute of Aging. He identified four other places and visited them one after another to investigate what was special about these places.

At first glance, the four could not have been more different: the island of Okinawa in Japan, the island of Ikaria in Greece, the Nicoya Peninsula in Costa Rica, and the community of Loma Linda in California. Buettner has since become an ambassador of healthy life and longevity, popularizing the concept of the blue zones and explaining what he discovered about these regions in books, conferences, and newspaper articles.

Beyond the superficial differences among the blue zones, he has found deeper affinities. He observed behavior and attitudes common to all the zones that are different from the behavior and attitudes typical in the rest of the world, and could explain the exceptional longevity of the blue zone inhabitants.

> Precisely because it was not a rich place, and because they were regularly threatened by invaders arriving from the sea, the inhabitants of Barbagia developed a strong sense of community and a strong culture of mutual aid.

Let us begin with Barbagia, the original blue zone in the center of Sardinia. History has not been kind to Barbagia. Quite the contrary, its name dates to Roman times, when Cicero described the region as a land of barbarians. The Romans, who controlled the coast of Sardinia but never managed to dominate the island's mountains, called its inhabitants *latroni ma strucati* (thieves with sheep skins). In ancient times, it was not a destination that anyone would consider suitable for retirement.

With a rough terrain of steep slopes and a Mediterranean forest, life there was not easy. Every plate of food required effort. Sheep needed to be tended and relatively infertile land had to be cultivated. The locals grew eggplants, zucchini, onions, and grapes, produced olive oil and pecorino cheese, and occasionally had meat. Precisely because it was not a rich place, and because they were regularly threatened by invaders arriving from the sea, the inhabitants of Barbagia developed a strong sense of community and a deeply rooted culture of mutual support.

This is a culture in which the family has more importance than in any modern urban society.

The blue zone of Barbagia has much in common with the island of Ikaria. Both are mountainous islands of the Mediterranean, where the land provides similar foods and where any displacement requires physical effort. Ikaria lacks natural harbors, and therefore, like Barbagia, has developed its own culture over the centuries, with few outside influences. This is a culture where the sense of community and family are also of great importance.

But Okinawa is a different case. First, it is in the Tropic of Cancer, which has a different climate than the Mediterranean islands; therefore, the locals have a different diet. With a location approximately the same distance from continental China as from the archipelago of Japan, it has been exposed to multiple external influences throughout its history. Since World War II, when the United States controlled Okinawa and left several military bases there, it has been exposed to Western influences. Despite these differences, the population of Okinawa has also maintained a lifestyle that allows its people to enjoy long, healthy lives.

According to the results of the Okinawa Centenarian Study, Okinawans seem to have special protection against the diseases associated with aging. Their arteries tend to remain in good condition up to an advanced age, with healthy levels of cholesterol and blood pressure that are not the result of any particular effort or diet. Their risk of breast and prostate cancer—two types of cancer often linked to hormonal factors—is 80 percent lower than the US population. They have half the hip fractures that Americans do and 20 percent of the whole of Japan, indicating greater bone health in older people. Those older than eighty-five have half the risk of Alzheimer's.

It is possible that the genetic profile of the population of Okinawa is partly responsible for their good health. In the previous chapter, we saw that the FOXO3 gene, associated with insulin activity, seems to benefit the people of Okinawa. The study of centenarians on the island has also pointed to low levels of inflammation thanks to a privileged immune system, specifically a variant of the HLA system that alleviates the inflammation reactions.

Even so, neither these nor other genes explain the differences in health and longevity between Okinawa and the rest of the world. There must be something more. The authors of the centenarian study highlight a diet without excess, low in sugars and calories, and faithful to the Confucian teaching of *Hara hachi bu*: "Eat until you are eight parts out of ten full." The population of Okinawa is the only one in the world that restricts calorie intake at mealtimes. It is not that they go hungry; rather, they refrain from eating until full or when they no longer have an appetite.

It should be noted that the population of Okinawa is physically active. It may come as no surprise that Okinawa is the birthplace of karate, a martial art that, despite its aggressive image portrayed by the film industry, has at its core basic principles of respect toward others, the avoidance of violence, and knowledge of oneself.

Diet and physical activity—there's nothing surprising here. But Buettner identified another common phenomenon among the centenarians of Okinawa that he interviewed. They call it *ikigai,* and it can be translated as "the reason to live" or, more modestly, "the reason to get up every morning." According to Japanese culture, each person must find *ikigai.* For one of the elders that Buettner interviewed, an eighty-eight-year-old fisherman, it was about going out every morning with his boat. For another, it was training every day and preparing for a decathlon at the age of eighty-four. For a woman who was 103 years old, it was spending afternoons talking and drinking tea with two friends with whom she had shared joys and sorrows since childhood. Every centenarian that Buettner interviewed in Okinawa had something that gave his or her life purpose.

BUETTNER IDENTIFIED ANOTHER COMMON PHENOMENON AMONG THE CENTENARIANS OF OKINAWA THAT HE INTERVIEWED. IT'S CALLED *IKIGAI* AND CAN BE TRANSLATED AS "A REASON FOR LIVING"...EVERY CENTENARIAN THAT BUETTNER INTERVIEWED IN OKINAWA HAD SOMETHING THAT GAVE HIS OR HER LIFE PURPOSE.

This, of course, does not prove that the *ikigai* is the cause of longevity. Being a subjective value, *ikigai* cannot be quantified, and its effects are difficult, if not impossible, to assess. We have all met people whose life was full of meaning and, regardless, died prematurely. We have also met people with low *ikigai* who lived many years. But regardless of the effect it may or may not have on longevity, one thing is certain: living with *ikigai* helps us to better enjoy the years we live.

There are two other blue zones we have not yet discussed: one in Costa Rica and the other in California. Each of them is unique. The one in Costa Rica is in the Nicoya Peninsula, which appears in maps as a little pinky finger venturing into the Pacific and, until a few years ago, was a world apart—away from highways. It is a poor region, but with a hospitable climate and generous nature that provides corn and tropical fruits in abundance.

There, Buettner found older people accustomed to working the land for food, whose religious beliefs bring them peace, as they believe that everything that happens is God's will and that tomorrow God will provide. This gives them hope for the future and relief from torments of the past. They maintain strong social bonds with family and neighbors. These are people who have little and do not need more.

The blue zone in California is more atypical. It is a community of the Seventh-day Adventist Church in the small town of Loma Linda, about fifty-nine miles east of Los Angeles. Since its foundation in the nineteenth century, the Adventist church has been teaching about health and community life. It prohibits tobacco and alcohol, limits the consumption of meat, and promotes a semi-vegetarian diet based on fruits, vegetables, cereals, and legumes. Its members maintain close ties within the community and devote Saturdays to church-related activities.

There is no need to be an Adventist to appreciate this style of life. Cornflakes, a breakfast cereal consumed today throughout the world, was created by John Harvey Kellogg, who was a Seventh-day Adventist. This is why the original brand name associated with this breakfast cereal is Kellogg's.

Because the Adventist lifestyle may prove instructive to those who do not share their religion, the National Institute of Health (NIH) has conducted several major studies on the Adventists. The studies have analyzed data from more than 150,000 people since the 1960s.

The results confirm that Adventists tend to live longer and in better health than most of us. In comparison to the rest of California's population, Adventist men live 7.3 years longer and women, 4.4. Mortality rate for cancer is 40 percent lower for Adventist men and 24 percent for women. And the mortality rate for coronary heart disease is 34 percent lower for men, though only 2 percent in women.

What lessons can we draw from these data? The most important and most obvious is that with a healthy lifestyle, we can live longer and better. This probably comes as no surprise. But it is worth taking a moment to clarify what that means. We explained in chapter 7 that health and longevity are regulated by genes. In this chapter, we added that they are regulated by lifestyle. The Loma Linda Adventists are not genetically different from the rest of the population of California. But they reach older ages in better health. Therefore, what many centenarians achieve thanks to a genetic inheritance, many of us can achieve by deciding how we should live our lives.

There is another less obvious, but just as important, lesson.

You may have noticed that the five blue zones described

above are islands, although not all seem like it. Sardinia, Ikaria and Okinawa are no doubt surrounded by sea. Nicoya Peninsula in Costa Rica is connected to the continent, but it has lived for centuries isolated from the rest of the country, and as a result developed its own culture and way of life. And although Interstate 10, which connects the whole southern US from California to Florida, crosses through Loma Linda, the Adventist community is a delimited one, like an island surrounded by land, with its own culture and values.

This means that the inhabitants of the blue zones do not choose to live as they do. They do not look after themselves because they care. They are just living as their community lives. We all do it, except we do not live on islands, but in communities with blurry borders. We eat what the people around us eat. We walk if others walk and drive our car where everyone else drives. We find it normal to live with stress if those around us also live with stress. We smoked when smoking was the norm and then stopped, or at least tried, when it stopped being socially accepted. There are endless examples.

The second lesson we can learn from these blue zones is that taking care of one's health cannot be considered an individual responsibility. It is a collective endeavor.

Pretending we can live a healthy lifestyle while everything

around us conspires against us can be a daunting task. It is understandable that those who attempt it fail, or if not, they feel socially excluded. In groups of adolescents where everyone smokes, the one who abstains is considered a weirdo. The same thing happens in groups that consume other drugs, or in those who practice risky sexual behavior, or drive recklessly, or gorge themselves on hypercaloric processed foods.

The behavior may seem different, but the phenomenon is the same. As you can see, we are social animals, and caring for our health is not what matters most to us. Feeling part of a community—being accepted and loved—is of higher value to us. That's why, if our family or our friends or the people we care about act in an unhealthy manner, it is easy for us to do the same. But the opposite is also true: if we are healthy, we help others be healthy.

If our health is important to us, we should ask ourselves if anything around us is conspiring to keep us from taking care of ourselves. It is a highly recommended exercise. Anyone who spends a few minutes with it ends up with a long list. It may be the routine of always being in the car, the vending machine where we get food every day, the habit of not eating a balanced breakfast, the demands of work robbing us of sleep, or the habit of watching TV until the early hours of the morning. The list is different for each person. But in modern urban societies, we are all exposed to thousands of stimuli that invite us to abuse our bodies.

At the same time, health is increasing in value. The number of people trying to switch to healthy diets and staying physically active is on the rise. As is the number of people who agree that smoking in public should be banned, people who try to reduce salt and sugar intake, people who accept and abide by laws and regulations to limit air pollution...This change of attitude towards our health within the community—which is no longer just a small island but rather the entire world, where we are all connected—is what might turn many of us into centenarians.

Five Regions of Extreme Longevity
Blue Zones studied by Dan Buettner

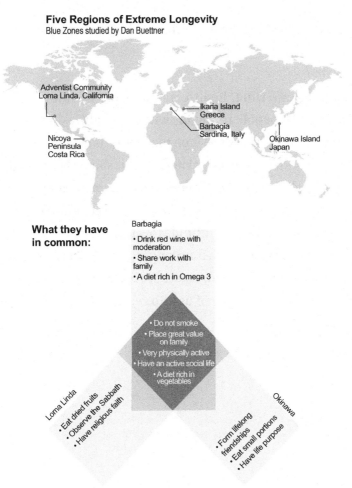

Adventist Community
Loma Linda, California

Nicoya —
Peninsula
Costa Rica

Ikaria Island
Greece

Barbagia
Sardinia, Italy

Okinawa Island
Japan

**What they have
in common:**

Barbagia
• Drink red wine with moderation
• Share work with family
• A diet rich in Omega 3

• Do not smoke
• Place great value on family
• Very physically active
• Have an active social life
• A diet rich in vegetables

Loma Linda
• Eat dried fruits
• Observe the Sabbath
• Have religious faith

Okinawa
• Form lifelong friendships
• Eat small portions
• Have life purpose

Source: "The Blue Zones" by Dan Buettner

WHY WOMEN LIVE LONGER

THE CONTROVERSIAL INFLUENCE OF SEX HORMONES ON LONGEVITY

By the middle of 2015, there were fifty-three supercentenarians—those living longer than 110 years—registered in the world. How many of them would you say were men and how many women? We will give you a hint: as the title of this chapter suggests, longevity is not evenly distributed between men and women. Another hint: if you have ever paid attention to life expectancy figures, you must have noticed that female life expectancy is higher than male life expectancy in any population. In Spain, for example, life expectancy at birth in the year 2015 was 85.7 years for women and 80.2 years for men. More than a five-year difference!

One might think that men are at greater risk of dying at an early age because they take more risks or because they take less care of themselves: more accidents, more alcohol, more tobacco, more lung cancer, more unhealthy foods, more heart attacks...And you might think that, when they reach a certain age, luck evens out. The data, however, disproves that theory. In Spain, the number of years that a woman is most likely to live—the age at which more women die, the statistical average—is eighty-eight years old. For men, it is eighty-four. There is still a four-year difference. If luck balances out after a certain age, this figure stays the same.

Let us get back to the supercentenarians; we asked how many of the fifty-three were men and how many were women.

Does anyone dare to take a guess? The answer is that only two were men and the remaining fifty-one were women.

When you stop to think about it, it is not so surprising that nature is so unfair. Men and women have different bodies; therefore, we must have equal rights. Compare a sample of a hundred men with one of a hundred women and you will find differences in weight, height, distribution of body fat, muscle mass, laxity of the ligaments, chromosomes in the nucleus of the cells, in the alcohol dehydrogenase enzyme that metabolizes alcohol more slowly in women...

In any biological parameter that you can think of, the truly strange thing would have been if, being so different in so many aspects, we were to be identical in life expectancy.

But what is the reason for this difference in life expectancy between men and women? A curious demographic study conducted in Korea on court eunuchs during the Chosun dynasty provides a possible explanation. The eunuchs were men deprived of testosterone, the male sex hormone. Castrated on purpose or by accident, they were employed for centuries in harems as servants or guards. In Korea, they were valued and enjoyed privileges, to the point that some children were deliberately castrated before reaching adolescence to gain access to the court.

Korea also has the Yang-Se-Gye-Bo, a document written in 1805 that is the only genealogical record of eunuch families in the world. It has birth and death dates, places of residence, rank in court, names of the wives and adopted children, and even the place of burial. A detailed analysis of this data has revealed that eunuchs in Korea lived an average of seventy years.

If seventy years does not seem like that long, consider that this data was from centuries ago—a time without antibiotics, operating rooms, emergency services, or public health. The average lifespan of men of a socioeconomic status similar to eunuchs was about fifty-three years. For the men of the royal family, it was forty-seven. Reaching seventy was nothing short of a tremendous feat.

An interesting fact: out of eighty eunuchs, three were centenarians. One even reached the age of 109 years old. Quite a Methuselah! If we recall that in the United States approximately 1 in every 6,000 people become a centenarian, the probability of living longer than a century was 220 times higher among the eunuchs of the Chosun dynasty than in modern societies.

This data seems to insinuate that testosterone is guilty of, or complicit in, the brevity of the male life. Other data points in the same direction. It has also been observed in dogs and rats that castration prolongs life. In men, elevated levels of testosterone contribute to the onset and progression of prostate cancer. The risk of coronary heart disease is higher in men than in women, especially before the age of fifty (although it has not been determined to what point testosterone is responsible for the difference; it might be completely innocent). In summary, with the data we have, we know that testosterone is suspect, but not guilty.

On the other hand, although women tend to live longer than men, it does not mean that there is something in the male body that is specifically harmful to them. The opposite could also be true: that there is something in the female body that is particularly beneficial, or something that women have in abundance and men do not. The most obvious candidate, of course, is estrogen, the main female sex hormone.

THE RISK OF CORONARY HEART DISEASE IS TWICE AS HIGH IN MEN THAN IN WOMEN, BUT IT HAS NOT BEEN CLARIFIED HOW TESTOSTERONE IS RESPONSIBLE FOR THAT DIFFERENCE, AND IT MIGHT EVEN BE COMPLETELY INNOCENT. WITH THE DATA THAT WE CURRENTLY HAVE, TESTOSTERONE IS SUSPECT, BUT NOT GUILTY.

The positive effects of estrogen are beyond doubt. Whether those positive effects outweigh the negative after menopause is under discussion.

It has been observed, for example, that a daily dose of estrogen lengthens the life of male mice. And, in women who reach menopause prematurely and take estrogen supplements, the risk of multiple age-related diseases— such as cardiovascular, neurodegenerative, osteoporosis, or cataracts—is reduced.

Which raises a question: how does estrogen achieve these beneficial effects? First, the female sex hormones have an antioxidant effect. They multiply the activity of genes that reduce oxidation and lower the amount of free radicals in the organism, so it is possible for the cell to accumulate less damage and tissues to stay healthy much longer. The male hormone testosterone, on the other hand, increases oxidative stress and elevates the quantity of free radicals, which in excess are harmful.

The female sex hormones have an antioxidant effect. They multiply the activity of genes that reduce oxidation and reduce the number of free radicals in the body.

Oxidative stress can shorten telomeres and damage DNA irreparably. Research conducted on the muscle progenitor cells has shown that, when too much damage is accumulated in the DNA, they enter a state of senescence and lose the ability to regenerate the tissue. That's why muscle injuries take longer to heal in older people than in young adults: the ability to repair the muscle is diminished. Anyone who has practiced physical activity for years has experienced this. There are pains that wear off in young people in just a few days, whereas in older people they might last weeks or months before disappearing. It also happens with wounds involving the skin, bone fractures, and damage to internal organs. With age, everything is worse.

But let us go back to estrogen. We said it has an antioxidant effect against free radicals. However, this is not its only anti-aging effect. It has also been observed to interact with the FOXO3 protein. This protein is what is called a transcription factor, meaning a protein that regulates the production of other proteins. It is like a big switch that controls much of what goes on inside the cells.

You may remember FOXO3. It appeared briefly in chapters 7 and 8, when we discussed the centenarians in Okinawa, Germany, and Hawaii. It's a protein that promotes longevity. An interesting detail is that FOXO3 is essential for the maintenance of hematopoietic progenitor cells, which renew the blood and are found in the bone marrow. And FOXO3 is also essential for the maintenance of neural progenitor cells that give rise to the various types of cells of the nervous system. In experiments in mice at least—and it is possible this also happens in people—these two types of stem cells are more abundant and more active in the female than in the male. This seems to support the idea that estrogen favors longevity.

And that is not all. Estrogen also activates an enzyme called telomerase. This enzyme is responsible for preserving the telomeres in the progenitor cells. Telomeres, already discussed in chapter 3, are the structures that protect the ends of the chromosomes. We compared them to the plastic bits at the end of shoelaces and said they get shorter throughout life. Therefore, thanks to estrogen, the progenitor cells can better preserve their telomeres and continue to function longer.

We have cited three possible effects of estrogen on longevity: free radicals, FOXO3, and telomeres. And the three converge in the progenitor cells, which are a type of cell responsible for the tissues that regenerate throughout life, as we explained in chapter 4.

Among the different types of progenitor cells, the telomeres and the various protective and harmful molecules, we have brought forth many protagonists to this story. They are all important, and it is possible that we may have confused you. But as you can see, the pieces of the puzzle are starting to fit together, and the protagonists of the different chapters are merging into the main story.

If estrogen is so beneficial, should we recommend a treatment for menopausal women when the body stops producing it? For years, it was thought to be a good idea, and hormone therapy was tremendously popular. It relieved the discomforts of menopause, such as hot flashes or vaginal dryness, and prevented subsequent health problems, such as osteoporosis and the risk of fractures. But today they have stopped prescribing it, and the use is limited to those women who are most likely to benefit from it.

It is important to know a few additional details to

understand why we changed our mind and who can still benefit from hormone therapy. This type of therapy usually combines two complementary hormones: estrogen and progesterone.

As its name indicates, estrogen regulates ovulation, causing estrus *(estro)* to produce *(gen)*. And progesterone is essential for pregnancy: in favor of *(pro)* gestation *(gesto)* to produce *(gen)*.

For this reason, during the reproductive life of a woman, estrogen predominates during the first half of the menstrual cycle, when the body is preparing to ovulate. And progesterone predominates during the second half, when the uterus is preparing to accept the fertilized egg. Because these two hormones are complementary and act in a coordinated manner, female hormone therapy often combines them.

Hormone therapy was once prescribed to hundreds of thousands of women throughout the world. Then a large clinical study that analyzed long-term effects detected that, along with the benefits, the therapy also entailed risks. It was a huge disappointment for the doctors who prescribed these, convinced they were helping their patients. But the data was unequivocal: the hormone therapy increased (very little, but increased) the risk of breast cancer, heart attack, and stroke.

Not that the increased risk was great. If 1,000 women undergo hormone therapy for five years continuously, four of them would have breast cancer that they may otherwise not have gotten. Four others will suffer a stroke. And an average of three and a half will suffer a coronary disease, such as a heart attack or angina. In contrast, three will avoid getting colorectal cancer that they may otherwise have gotten. And two and a half will avoid a hip fracture. When you mix all these statistical figures in the blender, the benefits and risks are compensated and there are no significant differences regarding the number of cancers or in total mortality. And if there are no significant benefits, there is no reason to recommend hormonal therapy indiscriminately to all women.

It was clarified later that progesterone increased cardio-vascular risk and estrogen reduced it. Would an estrogen therapy without progesterone be better? Estrogen, as we have said before, has an antioxidant effect. It preserves the telomeres of the stem cells and enhances the FOXO3 protein that protects against aging. At first glance, it may seem like the good guy of the story. However, when you break down the balance between hormones, estrogen favors abnormal growths in the tissues inside the uterus. Furthermore, it is responsible for the increased risk of breast cancer.

So what has become of hormone therapy today? It continues to be prescribed, when appropriate, to alleviate the symptoms of menopause that cause women great discomfort. In these cases, it is recommended to take the minimum effective dose and not to prolong the treatment longer than necessary.

Also, it is assessed in which cases the benefits likely outweigh the risks. For example, if a person has osteoporosis, estrogen can limit the loss of bone mass. In a family with a history of colon cancer but not of breast cancer, hormone therapy can reduce the overall risk of cancer. Or if a patient has the uterus removed, it may be appropriate to recommend estrogen therapy without progesterone.

It is also prescribed as a long-term treatment for women who experience premature menopause; otherwise, they would be more vulnerable to serious health problems such as coronary heart disease, osteoporosis, depression, or Parkinson's.

We are not telling you all this because we are trying to give you a crash course in hormone therapy, but because the estrogen story has an instructive lesson for those interested in the science of long life.

It seemed like the perfect anti-aging therapy for women. This is a simple pill that, taken once a day, would prolong the state of health of the reproductive stage well beyond menopause, maintaining the body of a young adult one birthday after another. And what remains of all this today? A therapy that tries to restore the natural functioning of the human body when it fails, as in cases of early menopause, but without trying to push the body beyond its limits when it is working well.

> Our body is extremely complex and, as one begins to manipulate a hormone or any other protein without considering all the other proteins with which it interacts, it is easy for them to provoke an issue we had not previously considered.

In hindsight, it was too good to be true. Our body is extremely complex and, when one begins to manipulate a hormone or protein without considering the other proteins that interact with it, without an overall view, it is easy to cause some type of issue not previously considered. As engineers would say—if it ain't broke, don't fix it.

Someone may promise you a simple and easy solution to staying young and strong and attractive, or some pill or potion or herb with nothing but benefits—except maybe the price—but no risk and no side effect. They may tell you, "Try it and you'll see how effective it is. All my clients are happy, and this celebrity takes it too." If someone comes to you with this speech, the lesson learned from hormone therapy tells us that it is best to take it with a grain of salt. I wish it were true. I wish there were a magic potion to promote long-term health. Unfortunately, there is not. The body is more complex than any pill that promises wonders. That is why it is so fascinating.

Female Life Expectancy Is Higher Than Male Life Expectancy around the World

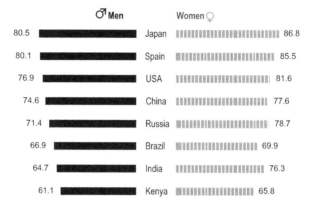

	♂ Men		Women ♀	
80.5		Japan		86.8
80.1		Spain		85.5
76.9		USA		81.6
74.6		China		77.6
71.4		Russia		78.7
66.9		Brazil		69.9
64.7		India		76.3
61.1		Kenya		65.8

Ranking of Countries with Longest Life Expectancy

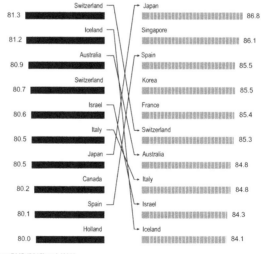

81.3	Switzerland	Japan		86.8
81.2	Iceland	Singapore		86.1
80.9	Australia	Spain		85.5
80.7	Switzerland	Korea		85.5
80.6	Israel	France		85.4
80.5	Italy	Switzerland		85.3
80.5	Japan	Australia		84.8
80.2	Canada	Italy		84.8
80.1	Spain	Israel		84.3
80.0	Holland	Iceland		84.1

Source: OMS (2015) and JAMA

The Differences Have Been Attributed Mainly to the Influence of Sex Hormones

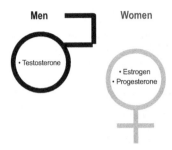

Hormone Treatments Have Risks as Well as Benefits

Risk of various diseases in postmenopausal women treated for 5 years with estrogen and progesterone vs. the untreated population

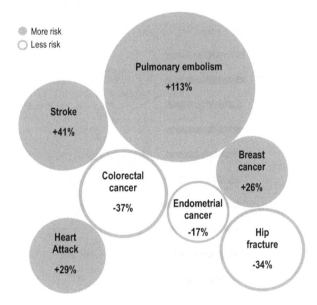

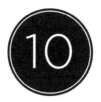

THE HAPPINESS CURVE

WHAT WE MEAN WHEN WE TALK ABOUT WELLBEING

Wouldn't you like to go back to being thirty years old, or even forty, and live a second youth? We could ask this question differently: are you happier now or when you were thirty years old?

Nearly all of us will answer yes to that first question. Of course, we would love to go back to being thirty years old and having our whole life ahead of us. But, if we are honest with ourselves, most of us will also answer affirmatively to the second question. Studies show that in developed countries, the feeling of subjective wellbeing increases with age.

Curious paradox: we want to be younger, although we

are happier when we are older. This suggests that current society may overvalue all that is associated with youth and underestimate all the good that comes with more advanced ages. The merits of being young are obvious, but rather hidden when we reach maturity. But they do exist. If you doubt it, and what we tell you here just seems like empty but well-meaning words, just wait until the end of the chapter. We hope to convince you of the positive side of growing older.

As you know, we live in a society that worships youth. We are exposed to a barrage of images of young bodies and faces. Models, actors, music stars, athletes...Nearly all of them are very successful.

There is economic logic behind it. We pay to see professional athletes at the peak of their career, not veterans' matches or competition among has-beens. A watchmaking business or a fashion designer would rather have one of these athletes—the image of success—as a spokesperson, or models that attract attention for their beauty, rather than someone that no one will notice. Youth sells; that is a fact. And if we want to sell watches or jeans or mobile phones or yogurt or anything, we will follow the logic of the system.

But we cannot blame the economic system for everything. This worship of youth in which we have immersed ourselves has a biological substrate. It appeals to our primate brain, which is attracted to images of human figures that promise fertility: young and beautiful bodies. It is no coincidence that the most ancient forms of prehistoric art are figures of Venus, and that ancient cultures worshipped young men of extreme beauty, such as Adonis in Greece or Tammuz in Babylon.

Whether we are comfortable admitting it or not, we are sexual animals with a powerful mating instinct developed over hundreds of millions of years of evolution. The rational brain of the human being, a newcomer in the history of life not more than a million years ago, can do little to overcome this instinct.

Whether due to economic pressure or biological imperatives, the result is that we live under the pressure of being, staying, or at least appearing, young. However, when you look at the evolution of happiness throughout life, this permanent desire to be young is unjustified.

This is an emerging field of research that, in recent years, has attracted a growing number of economists and psychologists concerned with the evaluation of the wellbeing of society beyond the classic economic indicators. Incidentally, this is a field of research of great prestige; its pioneer, Angus Deaton, was awarded the Nobel Memorial Prize in Economic Sciences in 2015 for his analysis of consumption, poverty, and welfare.

The results of his research contradict the classical view of the seven ages of life, whereby we are on the rise during the first half, we reach our peak at the adult stage, and then we experience a progressive decline towards old age until death. Interestingly, studies on happiness conducted in recent years draw a curve that is inverted in developed countries. This is a curve that, instead of having the form of an arch, first with a rise and then with a descent, is U-shaped. First it goes down, and then it goes up.

We begin our adult life, around the age of twenty, with high levels of happiness. It gradually declines in the following years, so slowly that we usually do not even realize it. We have obligations, concerns, and stress. We experience increasing family-related and work-related stress. We get to our lowest point between the ages of forty and fifty-five, give or take a few years depending on the person. There is a point of change popularly known as a midlife crisis. Then we begin to soar as we learn to shed weight, avoid trivial concerns, and value what we care about the most. This is the happiness curve of a typical person in Spain or in any other developed economy.

One might think at first glance that this curve is partly related to the economic situation of each person. If the income is not enough to provide when we are young, it is normal to experience economic hardship, problems paying the bills, and worry. If we find ourselves in a more stable professional situation later, we can be calmer and enjoy life more fully.

But studies on happiness show that this U-shaped curve is largely independent of external factors such as income or whether a person has children or a job. The curve is more dependent on internal attitudes.

WE BEGIN ADULTHOOD WITH HIGH LEVELS OF HAPPINESS. IT GRADUALLY DECLINES IN THE FOLLOWING YEARS. WE ARRIVE AT THE LOWEST POINT BETWEEN THE AGES OF FORTY AND FIFTY-FIVE. THEN WE BEGIN TO SOAR AS WE LEARN TO SHED WEIGHT, AVOID TRIVIAL CONCERNS, AND VALUE WHAT WE CARE ABOUT THE MOST.

How we each decide to live our lives and relate to the world confirms the adage that money does not buy happiness.

In fact, the topic is only partially true. When analyzing data from populations around the world, as did Angus Deaton, the Nobel recipient mentioned earlier, it is observed that people living in rich countries are, overall, happier than those in poor countries. We sometimes admire the smile of African children and wonder how they can be happy with so little when we hear their stories of survival, but these smiles are not habitual. Sub-Saharan Africa is the region of the world with the lowest recorded levels of happiness, across all age groups.

In countries with lower poverty rates, citizens go through economic difficulties throughout their lives and never stop worrying about the future. For citizens living in countries like Latin America or the former Soviet Union, the curve appears not in a U shape, but in a progressive decline in happiness throughout their lives. So, which is it? Does money buy happiness or not? What these studies tell us is that poverty is a cause for unhappiness. But, from the moment their basic needs are covered and they are not permanently worried about the future, people find that having more money will not make them any happier.

Those who have much, on the whole, are not happier than those who have enough. The opposite can happen. The more options there are to choose from, the harder it is to know what we want. We have all experienced it when looking at a restaurant menu with too many options, or choosing what music to listen to, or buying clothes. So, when we have access to all kinds of goods and distractions, we devote more time to stimuli that is nice but not important. And we end up finding it much more difficult to focus on what is truly fulfilling and to be clear about our priorities.

Maybe by now you are wondering what all this has to do

with the science of a long life. You will find the answer in this last word: priorities. It is to discover what really matters to us.

Studies on the evolution of happiness throughout life identify three different dimensions of wellbeing. One is hedonic wellbeing (or experiential wellbeing, as some researchers prefer to call it), which is a short-term feeling and describes the day-to-day state of mind. It is the type of wellbeing we experience when we feel happy or content, or that we stop feeling when we are sad, angry, or worried. However, immediate moods do not reflect all the nuances of happiness. That is why there are people that, without having a cheerful character, feel perfectly happy. Or people who, appearing more cheerful, are not so happy.

There is, on the other hand, a deeper, more stable level of wellbeing, which fluctuates slightly from one day to another. We call it evaluative wellbeing. It describes each person's assessment of their own life. This is whether they are satisfied with their life or if they would rather live another way.

If hedonic wellbeing is the waves on the surface, hectic one day and calm the next, evaluative wellbeing is the undercurrent. Waves, just like moods, depend on external influences such as the wind or pressure. The undercurrent depends more on the internal state of each person—their mood at an intimate level.

These two types of wellbeing, hedonic and evaluative, do not always go together. For example, people who live with children at home often express higher levels of anger and stress than people without children. But when asked to assess their level of satisfaction with their life—in other words, their evaluative wellbeing—they often score higher than people without children.

When hedonic wellbeing is broken down into different types of basic emotions, such as Angus Deaton did in his study with more than 340,000 participants, it confirms that the majority of people tend to feel better as years go by.

Positive emotions such as happiness and enjoyment follow the U-shaped curve we described earlier. What is observed with negative emotions is even more interesting. Anger follows a downward slope, with a maximum level at the age of twenty and a progressive and uninterrupted descent into old age. Stress begins at a high level, goes up until around the age of twenty-five, and then slopes downward. Worry is maintained at high levels until around the age of fifty before it starts to go down.

Therefore, in these three cases—anger, stress, and worry—

the older we get, the less negativity we have. If you are the type of person that feels that each birthday is a small annual torture—something you must go through, hoping that no one finds out—those are three good arguments to reconsider this point of view.

The only negative emotion that does not tend to decline with age is sadness. But neither does it increase. Though at an individual level it has its ups and downs according to the vicissitudes of life, when we add the population data, sadness remains stable, without significant level changes throughout life.

We have mentioned before that studies have identified three dimensions of wellbeing, but you might have noticed that we only mentioned two: hedonic and evaluative. We have saved the most important for last: the eudaimonic dimension.

The word comes from Greek philosophy. It refers to happiness as a state of fulfillment different from pleasure. Aristotle was the first to reflect deeply on the difference between pleasure and happiness, and his legacy has traversed the whole history of Western thought, from Christianity to modern science. Aristotle argued that to achieve happiness, human beings must act according to the natural order. Christianity expressed it in terms of moral law, conforming to the commandments of God. In the eighteenth century, Kant argued that human beings should be guided by a sense of duty. And now in the twenty-first century, scientific studies reflect the idea that the deepest form of wellbeing is linked to the meaning of life. They are nuances around the same central idea.

Scientific studies revealed that people who achieve eudaimonic wellness are those who find meaning in life, a mission, something worth living for.

Of course, this wellbeing is not exclusive to Western culture. It is a product of the human brain that can take root in any culture. If you remember in chapter 8, where we discussed the centenarians of the island of Okinawa, eudaimonic wellness is the same thing as *ikigai*: the reason to get up every morning.

> Finding a purpose in life is essential to growing old, healthy and continuing to enjoy life at advanced ages. Not just because it sounds nice. It's what the data shows.

Not everyone can find a reason to get up every morning. But to find meaning in life is essential to growing old, healthy and continuing to find joy at advanced ages. Not just because it sounds nice. This is what the data shows. Data such as that from the ELSA (English Longitudinal Study of Aging), which involved more than 9,000 volunteers who had an average age of sixty-five at the start of the research and were followed for about eight-and-a-half years. They were asked, among other things, about their level of psychological wellbeing in a survey that included the assessment of their life purpose or their degree of fulfillment.

Inevitably, when studying a large group of sixty-five-year-old people, some tend to die within the following years. What the ELSA study revealed is that, among 25 percent of participants who experienced the highest level of eudaimonic wellbeing, 9 percent died throughout the study. Among the 25 percent who had the lowest level of eudaimonic wellbeing, more than triple the participants died: 29 percent.

All variables were analyzed to evaluate their potential influence. Whether it was related to educational level, income, mood at the beginning of the study, physical activity, consumption of alcohol...After discarding all imaginable variables, the protective effect of eudaimonic wellbeing was maintained, with a 30 percent reduction in the risk of death over the next eight and a half years in a population of sixty-five-year-olds.

For those brought up in the era of molecular biology, convinced that everything that happens in the human body has a biochemical explanation, this great effect of the eudaimonic wellbeing may seem implausible. It is surely a controversial effect, but the ELSA is not the only one to have detected it.

In the United States, the same effect was observed in a group of people who were eighty-four years old at the beginning of the study. They underwent an annual and psychological checkup in the following years and got an autopsy upon their death—which occurred at an average age of ninety. The autopsy revealed which of them had lesions in the brain caused by a stroke. The first result showed that approximately half of people who had suffered strokes had not been diagnosed the moment it occurred. But the most interesting result appeared when the risk of stroke was associated with eudaimonic wellness; those who more intentionally expressed to be living a life with purpose at the age of eighty-four had a 44 percent lower risk of having a stroke. Just as in the ELSA, the effect remained when variables such as blood pressure, physical activity, and depression were ruled out.

A biochemical explanation has not been found for this protective effect of eudaimonic wellbeing, but it does not mean it does not exist. The explanation could be related to cortisol, a hormone released in stressful situations and that has harmful effects on the body, such as the fat metabolism and the immune system. Or it could be related to inflammation, which also has harmful effects that are reduced in situations of emotional wellbeing. Whatever the mechanism, the data is clear: having a purpose in life is good for your health.

At this point, some of you are probably saying, "Thanks for the advice, gentlemen, but I don't need it. I have not had a sense of mission in my life, and I have been just fine. Besides, if I have not yet found clear purpose, I don't see how I could do it now."

It is a perfectly legitimate position, of course. Everyone is free to live their lives as they see fit. But if someone feels devoid of this sense of purpose and is searching for *ikigai* but not sure how to find it, here are two examples that may prove useful.

These are examples of two people who managed major institutions in the United States. They were very influential and respected—admired, even—and when they reached the age of seventy, they were out of work. They were forced into retirement. It was a shock for both. One had been a political leader; the other had managed an antiquities museum. From one day to the next, they were left with nothing to do. One sank. Everything that had given meaning to his life—feeling valued, having social success, sensing the power to open any door and be welcomed—all of that vanished. Where he had once found meaning, now there was nothing. He died a few years later.

The other resurfaced. Once the initial shock had passed, he started an organization that educated underprivileged children. He stopped caring about what he had done up until then and started caring again about what he could do in the future. Today, he is still active and hopeful.

The essential difference between these two people, if you stop and think about it, is the future. It is the prospect of a future, the sense of having a mission, a purpose in life, our *ikigai*—or as some prefer to call it, the result of the difference and not the cause.

The essential difference is that the first man valued himself in terms of how others valued him. He had done what was expected of him, and he had done it well. But he did not have his own priorities; his priorities were those of others. In a way, he had lived dominated by social norms and by the expectations of others.

The second man, however, cared little about what others thought. He did not do what was expected of him, but what he felt he should do: museum manager for a time and then mine deactivation. Sometimes he coincided with what others expected, and sometimes it mattered little to him. His main motivation was not to please, though of course he enjoyed being valued. His motivation was internal. This allowed him to set his own priorities, not to let himself be swayed by social norms, and to find a new purpose in life, which brings us back to the curve of happiness and to the subject of how to live a long life, enjoying it until the very end.

Achieving eudaimonic wellbeing, as we have seen, requires a person be able to define their priorities. This is much more than having something to do; it is about knowing what we want to spend the rest of our time doing in this world.

When we have no priorities, we allow ourselves to be swayed by the environment. From the moment we know what our priorities are, we no longer allow ourselves to be dominated. It is not easy, since prioritizing requires renouncing activities and opportunities that we feel tempted to accept, such as attending events we are invited to, accepting extra work, or indulging more trivial distractions like watching a TV show or lingering on social networks. The list is long. And it is personal and non-transferable.

As no two people are the same, because we are all unique in our way, priorities may not be the same for everyone. What fulfills one person seems inconsequential to another. That is why no one can tell us what should be more important for us—it is something we must discover ourselves. And we can only find out what it is if we stop caring about what others think, what they will say, or whether they will compliment or criticize us. If we strive to conform to social norms—norms which we have already seen worship the beauty of youth—then we are doomed to misery. As much as science has advanced, we will not look twenty years old when we are eighty. And even if we could, newer generations would still be there to remind us that we are not equal. Only if we accept ourselves as we are, without worrying excessively about what others think, can we reach eudaimonic wellbeing, which is the true wellbeing.

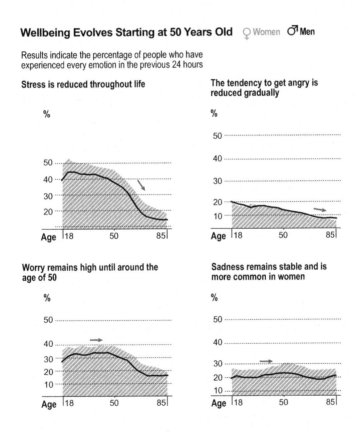

Wellbeing Evolves Starting at 50 Years Old ♀ Women ♂ Men

Results indicate the percentage of people who have experienced every emotion in the previous 24 hours

Stress is reduced throughout life

The tendency to get angry is reduced gradually

Worry remains high until around the age of 50

Sadness remains stable and is more common in women

The feeling of enjoyment increases after 50 years old

The feeling of happiness decreases until the age of 50, then it goes back up

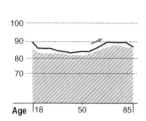

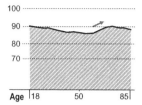

Overall wellbeing has the lowest levels of life around the age of 50, and then it goes back up. It is higher in women than in men

Rating on a scale of 0 to 10 (population mean)

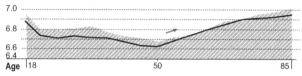

Results of a study led by the Nobel laureate Angus Deaton made in USA in 2008 with the data of 340,847 people

Source: PNAS

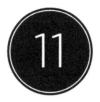

FROM PYRAMIDS TO SKYSCRAPERS

HOW LONG WE COULD LIVE: THE NEW DEMOGRAPHIC REVOLUTION

As much as we might accept the passage of time at the individual level and achieve a good level of eudaimonic wellbeing, the truth is that we still do not accept the aging process at a social level. That is no country for old men, as Yeats said in one of his poems about the passage of time (which inspired the title of a novel by Cormac McCarthy, which in turn inspired a movie by the Coen brothers— nothing comes from nothing!). But Yeats fell short. The reality is that it is no *world* for the old.

This demonstrates how absurd we have become as human beings. We all strive to live longer and better with scientific studies, self-care products, books like the one you have in your hands, and our own individual efforts—but then, when we manage to live longer, we all take part in rejecting older people. Little by little, we leave them without work, without social relevance, without autonomy, without company.

> We all strive to live longer and better, with scientific studies and self-care products, but then when we manage to live longer, we all take part in rejecting older people.

Faced with this contradiction, one might wonder if we truly want to live longer. Not just selfishly wishing it for ourselves, but also for the whole of humanity. Because living a longer life but not a fuller one may not be worth it. If we are honest with ourselves, we must recognize that we have a problem—an unresolved problem.

We have created it with the great advances of science and medicine in the last century and a half. It is a side effect, if you will. Seen this way, it is a very recent phenomenon in the history of humanity—a story that is over twenty-thousand centuries old, to which we have yet to adapt.

The fact is that we are witnessing an unprecedented increase in life expectancy in the world, in both rich and poor countries. Globally, life expectancy has increased at a rate of three years per decade over the past decades. It has done so consistently, and for now, there is no indication that this increase is going to slow down, in the short or medium terms. In 1990, the average life expectancy at birth was sixty-five years and four months; in 2013, it had risen to seventy years old and six months. If we continue at this rate, around the year 2040—it is not that far away; it is like the day after tomorrow—life expectancy at birth will have reached the age of eighty for the whole of humanity.

So far, these are global figures, impersonal and abstract. If we go more into detail, we will have a better understanding of their effect upon us. First detail: by ages. Life expectancy has historically increased because infant mortality has been reduced and, at a lesser rate, mortality in young adults. With more vaccines, better hygiene, new medicines, fewer accidents, and less malnutrition, the prospects of enjoying a long life and seeing the birth of our great-grandchildren have multiplied.

But we are now witnessing a new phenomenon. Not only is mortality reduced among the very young, but also among older people. And it is happening at a rate never seen in the history of mankind. In rich countries, the life expectancy of a sixty-year-old person has increased three years in two decades. Both in men and women. Topping the ranking is the female population of Japan, with a sustained increase of 0.24 years each year between 1990 and

2011. This means that, for every day that passes, Japanese women over sixty years of age earn, on average, six hours of life. And for every year, they earn three months. Not bad, right? Japan is not a unique case; it is simply the most extreme. The same phenomenon is observed in all the developed economies of the world. In the United Kingdom, for example, men have won 0.21 years every year, or about five hours each day, in the same two decades. In Australia, it is the same. In New Zealand, it is even more.

The result is that today, when people reach eighty years of age, they still tend to have a long road ahead. Not everyone, of course. We all know that an eighty-year-old, or even younger, may have poor health. But, if they are healthy, there is no reason to consider them old, beyond the prejudice that eighty means being old.

This bias might have been reasonable a generation ago. But it no longer conforms to the new reality of improved health and increased survival among older people. The new reality is that, in developed countries, an eighty-year-old man now has an average life expectancy of nine years, and a woman, of eleven. Therefore, if they are in good health, they still have many years ahead—more than 10 percent of their life. Is anyone willing to give up enjoying 10 percent of their life just because there is social pressure that leads one to think that if one is eighty years old, or whatever the number, one should feel old?

At the same time, we continue to witness the gradual reduction of premature deaths among children, adolescents, and young adults. This reduction is the basis of what is termed the demographic transition, which first describes a decline of mortality and then of births when moving from a preindustrial economy to a modern economy. With advances in prevention and medical treatment, infant and juvenile mortality from diseases have been virtually eradicated in rich countries, and mortality from accidents has been reduced to a minimum. Just two centuries ago, it was normal for some of the children of a family to die during childhood. Today, we no longer consider it normal. Today, it is unacceptable, and whenever it happens, it is a drama. This, while it may not seem so at first glance, also has to do with the science of long life. It is related because it has irreversibly upset the population pyramids. A population pyramid, let us remember, is a chart that describes population by age group. At the base are the newborns, and in the highest part, the elderly. That is why, in a country in which premature deaths occur at all ages, the number of people gets smaller as the age increases, and the graph narrows from the base to the top. Thus, the shape of the graph has been compared to a pyramid.

But what will happen if you remove the premature mortality of children and adolescents? Simply, each floor will be as wide as the previous one, and instead of a pyramid there will be a tower.

And what will happen next if we eliminate mortality in the adult population—for example, deaths from heart attacks that could have been prevented, or tobacco-related cancer, or traffic accidents? The tower will be increasingly consistent because all the floors will be equally wide, not only up to the ages of twenty or thirty but up to sixty or seventy.

And what will happen in the upper floors if we consider that life expectancy is increasing rapidly in those over sixty, as we have previously explained? Exactly what we are seeing now: that the tower is gaining height, and the pyramid becomes a skyscraper.

It is a curious metaphor, don't you think? In ancient times, we had pyramids, and now we have skyscrapers, both in architecture and demography. We don't know what height it will reach, because the building is still in construction. It continues to grow, year after year. Each year, there are more and more tenants living on the 100th floor, the one with the centenarians. And we know from Jeanne Calment that it is not impossible to reach 122—though, for now, there is no need for more rooms.

It might be fun to play "The Rear Window" and amuse ourselves by watching what happens on the higher floors. We do not have a skyscraper of equal angles and cubic forms like the Twin Towers used to be. This would mean that everyone would reach the maximum age possible. It may seem like an ideal target from a public health point of view, but it may not be from a psychological viewpoint, since we would know in advance how long we are going to live.

What we see is more like the Empire State Building or the Agbar Tower in Barcelona. A building that rises in a straight line and then begins to narrow when it reaches the highest floors.

This happens because we have managed to avoid premature mortality, which has been one of the major successes in the history of humanity, but no one has worried about avoiding premature aging. We didn't know it could be avoided, let alone how to do it. Now we are starting to learn how, as we explain in the next chapters. The result is that between the floors seventy and eighty, our skyscraper begins to narrow. Later, as it gains height, it becomes increasingly thin. And above the 120th floor, there is only sky.

Speaking of architecture, allow us to tell you the story of I. M. Pei, the architect who built the Louvre Pyramid. He was born in China in 1917 and lost his mother to cancer when he was thirteen years old. At eighteen, he came to the United States to study architecture; later, he met the legendary Le Corbusier at the Massachusetts Institute of Technology, which marked him deeply. He moved to

New York to begin his career and ended up becoming one of the most important architects of the second half of the twentieth century. While he no longer goes to his office every day, Pei has never truly retired. At almost one hundred years of age, he is still active and engaged. Speaking with him, one is infused with his enthusiasm. He is still as curious as a child, eager to learn, and filled with intellectual restlessness. During his world travels, he has always observed buildings and cities like a doctor might observe the human body. To see how they are built, how they work, how they are integrated in the environment, the nuances of light, the texture of the material, the harmony of shapes...In short, he sees what others are missing. He sees the complete architectural system, in all its complexity, and enjoys it as one would enjoy a work of art.

We tell you this story because it might be helpful to learn how Pei can maintain such vitality at his age. Is it an isolated case, or is there something there that can guide us? When one has built innovative buildings and landmarks and has been both applauded with devotion and criticized vehemently, one learns to not pay too much attention to criticism or praise, and to simply do what one believes in. What is special about Pei—just like the man who went from managing a museum to deactivating mines—is his attitude. It is an inner conviction that he does what he should and he does it because he wants to, away from seeing a world that conforms to social stereotypes. He does not care if the world sees centenarians as old. Pei lives his life his way. *My way*, as Sinatra sang. And he feels great.

Let us now return to our skyscrapers and continue our game of "The Rear Window." The most interesting things will be found on the intermediate floors, more or less between the twentieth and seventieth floors, which is the part of the building where adults live. Traditionally, students used up the floors to the twentieth, families with children went up to the twenty-fifth floor, people who worked up to the fortieth floor, and the retirees settled on the sixty-fifth floor and above.

But in modern urban societies worldwide, this distribution is shifting upwards. Students now reach the thirtieth floor. It is hard to find families with children there, because almost all of them have moved up to the thirty-fifth or fortieth floor.

This move changes our perception about aging. Think about the ones who are thirty years old today. Do you see them more as youths in training or leaders capable of leading? Well, at thirty, Napoleon was the leader of France. The Beatles completed their entire work before the age of thirty. And George Lucas wrote *Star Wars* at thirty-two. Now think of people who are forty. A generation ago, they were in their full professional maturity; now, they are more often seen as people whose careers are just taking off.

And now think of those that are sixty-five. These have not changed that much. Sixty-five is still, in many countries, the age of retirement. But look at the whole building. Floor sixty-five in a building of more than one hundred floors: do you think that floor is too high? The truth is that it is closer to the middle than the rooftop.

This skyscraper, which represents all of society, is like a great community of neighbors. We all must organize ourselves and resolve our issues. It is an enormous community, and we do not know each other personally. But we must help our neighbor the day he needs it if we hope to have someone willing to help us when we need it someday.

Now we have the community organized in thirds. In the lower third, more or less up to the thirtieth floor, are the children and young adults that are still developing. In the middle third, up to the sixty-fifth or seventieth floor, are those that strive to make everything work: those that support the education of the young, care for the elderly, and obtain everything they need themselves. In the upper third live the elderly who, in most cases, have stopped working for the community.

What will happen if the building gains height? We have seen that longevity is increasing. What if we raise the developmental age and push back the working age at the same time? It is basic math—a question of proportions. What will happen is that the proportion of people who contribute to the community compared to the total number of neighbors in the building will be reduced.

You can work your rear end off. In fact, in many countries, we are seeing that those who have work sometimes endure draconian conditions to support their children and their elders. But the inevitable consequence is that the whole community degrades.

Take, for example, health care costs. With more seniors, costs are destined to increase. But these costs can hardly be met if the proportion of working people is reduced relative to the total population. This can lead us to a situation in which, after prolonging human life and congratulating ourselves on the spectacular success of science and medicine, we find that we have no resources to care for the elderly and cannot guarantee a good quality of life at an advanced age.

How do we resolve this problem? There is no other solution than to enable everyone to contribute to the community to the best of their abilities. This means tearing down the dynamic that when one reaches the age of sixty-five, one ceases to be a member of an active population and becomes part a passive population.

There are many ways to continue contributing. One that is particularly unpopular in Europe is delaying the retirement age.

IN THE LOWER THIRD, MORE OR LESS UP TO THE THIRTIETH FLOOR, ARE THE CHILDREN AND YOUNG ADULTS…IN THE MIDDLE THIRD, UP TO THE SIXTY-FIFTH OR SEVENTIETH FLOOR, ARE THOSE WHO STRIVE TO MAKE THINGS WORK… IN THE UPPER THIRD LIVE THE ELDERLY WHO, IN MOST CASES, HAVE STOPPED WORKING FOR THE COMMUNITY.

Does it make sense that a person who is in full physical and intellectual form, who also has the value of experience, should be forced to retire? Do you not think it is a ridiculous waste of human capital?

If you do not enjoy work and delaying retirement seems unacceptable to you, there are other ways to contribute to the community. The most popular, and much more widespread, is to help care for the grandchildren. Another one is to help take care of the elderly, or to get involved in social work, like the man who helped educate under-privileged children, or as someone participating in an

NGO. These are all valid. What is not sustainable is to do nothing.

Possibly, right now some of you are thinking, "I don't like this book anymore. After so many years working, I have earned the right to a quiet retirement. The last thing I need are two guys telling me what I need to do!" You are right. If you do not want to do anything, we are no one to tell you what you should do.

> Do not stay locked at home just because you have retired and are treated as a passive population, like some old geezer who no longer has anything valuable to provide. Yes, you do.

But if there is anything that motivates you, something that you think might be worth getting into, for yourself or others, do like the architect Pei. Do not stay locked at home just because you have retired and are treated as a passive population, like some old geezer who no longer has anything valuable to provide. Yes, you do. We can all contribute to the community so long as we are healthy. And if you find something worth waking up for every morning—if you find your *ikigai*—you will see that doing something for others, even if effort is involved, does not hurt you but rather enriches you.

The Evolution of the Population Pyramids

Men ♂ ♀ Women

SOCIETIES OF THE PAST

With a high premature mortality, the population is reduced in each age

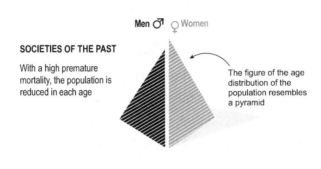

The figure of the age distribution of the population resembles a pyramid

CURRENT SOCIETIES

With less infant mortality, birth is reduced

The reduction of the elderly population does not begin to be appreciated significantly until around the age of 50

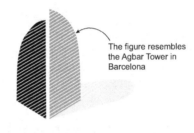

The figure resembles the Agbar Tower in Barcelona

FUTURE SOCIETIES

Practically without premature mortality

The tower gains height thanks to increased longevity

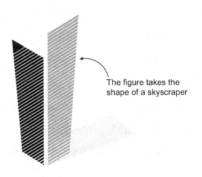

The figure takes the shape of a skyscraper

THE TREE OF LIFE

THE LAW OF NATURE: IF YOU DON'T USE IT, YOU LOSE IT

We began by telling you about the cells that make up the human body and the wonders that take place inside (chapter 3). We then discussed the tissues and organs formed by these cells, and how they degrade and renew (chapters 4 and 6). We went on to widen our focus as we talked about the human body as a unit (chapters 7 to 10). Then, we widened the focus even more to talk about how humans relate to each other (chapter 11).

We have traveled from the smallest scale of life to the largest; it is possible that you have noticed repeating patterns. The easiest pattern to see is in architecture: how the system is built. Cells interact with each other and form tissues and organs. The tissues and organs interact and form the human body. Human beings interact and form communities. Communities interact and form the whole of humanity. And, if you want to go further still, the human species interacts with other species and forms the biosphere. In our little planet, the journey ends there for now.

The same structure, if you look closely, can be observed in trees. The trunk is divided into branches, the branches into smaller branches, and those smaller branches into twigs, and so on. The same structure is repeated in our circulatory system. The big aorta artery bifurcates into minor arteries. These, in turn, break off into smaller arteries. Then come the arterioles, and then the capillaries. This makes it possible for the blood to get to the end of its trajectory, charged with oxygen and nutrients, to all corners of the human body.

This type of structure in which a same pattern repeats at different scales is what we call a fractal. The idea of fractals comes from mathematics. Benoît Mandelbrot, who invented the word and popularized the concept, was also the oldest person to obtain a tenure post in the three centuries of history of Yale University. They hired him at the age of seventy-five. This is another example of a person who remained active while having something to contribute.

Mandelbrot was a remarkable mathematician. He was

fascinated by the beauty of shapes and the elegance of formulas, and he had an insatiable curiosity. After graduating in mathematics, he majored in aeronautics, taught economics at Harvard University, and worked most of his career as a researcher for IBM.

During his career at IBM, he used computers and printers to convert mathematical formulas into images. If we want to print a straight line, for example, simply send the printer a formula for a straight line. But Mandelbrot was devoted to exploring more complex formulas. When he sent a formula to print, he did not know what the result would be. He did not know what images he would get until the printer gave him the answer.

The results he achieved were spectacular and something never seen before. He created images that no one had imagined. If they looked at any part of the image, they would see the same as if they were looking at the whole image. If they focused on a smaller part, they still saw the same thing. If they looked with a magnifying glass, it was still the same. The same forms would repeat at all scales to the microscopic infinite.

Fractals, it would soon be learned, are not exclusive to mathematics. They are everywhere in nature. They are in the branches and in the roots of the trees; in snowflakes, where water molecules organize themselves to form stars with bifurcating branches. In clouds, where the shapes are similar at all scales—it is hard to know the actual size from a photo of a cloud fragment. It is in the distribution of stars in galaxies and galaxies in the universe. Fractals are—one of the most classic examples—in the elegant complexity of the leaves of the Romanesco broccoli. They are in the brilliance of lightning and the waves of the ocean. And they are, as we have seen, in the human body—in the circulatory tree and the rough surface of the brain, among many other examples.

So far, these are all examples of architecture, which are the easiest to see. They are still images that allow us to stop and contemplate how nature is built. Besides the still images, fractals also offer movies, in examples not only of how they are built but also how they work. In how the same processes are repeated again and again at different scales.

Look at evolution, which is the basic process that organizes life on Earth. One generation after another reproduces the same pattern of creation, copy, and destruction; creation, copy, and destruction; creation, copy, and destruction, time after time. Take Earth billions of years ago, when living beings had only a single cell and the first animal had not yet been born; or 100 million years ago, in the dinosaur era; or now in the era of humans. The process is the same even if the scale is different. The biosphere is not the same today as it was billions of years ago, and not just because we humans have transformed. Evolution itself has transformed one generation after another, one species after another, one ecosystem after another. That is how life operates on a large scale: with fractal tenacity.

It also works on a small scale. Going back to the human body, the same pattern is observed at the scale of cells, tissues, the body, and the community. In chapters 7 and 8, we discussed how centenarians tend to be active people. This is at the scale of the organism. But if we look at smaller scales, the same thing happens. If we do not exercise the heart and lungs, we lose cardiorespiratory fitness. If we do not challenge the brain, it stagnates. You might have found this out already if you play piano or chess or any other activity that requires a certain mental agility. When we stop practicing, we lose skills.

We can go to even smaller scales and see the same thing. A tissue that is not worked is a tissue that is degraded, just as muscles atrophy when we do not work them. Or just like the astronauts who go to space: when they come back to Earth, their bones are more fragile after months of not having to support the weight of the body. This happens even with cells, which must be removed once they stop working, if you remember chapter 4.

Why does this happen? Would it not be better, when a cell or a tissue or an entire body stops working, to let it rest? Maybe it would be better from our point of view as primates, but in nature, everyone must earn their keep. The tiger cannot afford to say, "This week I do not feel like hunting, so I am going to take a break." If he does not hunt, he does not eat. If he does not eat, it is goodbye.

It is a general law: there is no vacation in nature. Evolution is guided by a logic of competition and selection, so that, over billions of years, the mechanisms of life have become highly efficient. Everything that is not used is lost. Of course, we humans have freed ourselves, in part, from the law of the jungle. We can take a vacation. We can fall ill and receive care. Spend a long, unproductive season without being removed from the system, unlike the tiger that stopped hunting. We can enjoy leisure: games when we are children and retirement when we are older. All of these have been major cultural achievements that we must preserve.

But the body that we are born into and in which we live is not only the product of culture. It is, above all, a work of nature. We can modify it to some extent with our actions—with what we eat, our lifestyle, interventional and cosmetic surgery, tattoos...In fact, we change it a little bit every day when we brush our teeth, cut our nails, take a drug, or put on shoes. But we cannot escape the fundamental law of nature that everything that is not used is lost.

> To keep our organs and tissues in good condition, we
> should keep them active...The question we face is: how
> is it possible to stay active with dwindling strength?

You see, the classic metaphor that describes the human body as a machine is incorrect. The perfect machine, as the cliché goes. Or the incredible machine, according to *National Geographic*. It is true that it is a highly sophisticated invention, capable of implausible feats. But it is not a machine. Think about that for a moment. Machines work well when new, but with use they become less efficient, and the more they are used, the more they wear down. With the human body, the opposite happens. Everything begins to fail when not used.

And, if we come back to the main question of how to live a long life and enjoy it, it raises a dilemma. We have seen that, to conserve our organs and tissues in good condition, we should keep them active. But as we get older, as we have seen in chapter 6, we tend to lose breathing capacity, muscle strength, sight, hearing, and one or two teeth.

BUT THE BODY THAT WE ARE BORN INTO AND IN WHICH
WE LIVE IS NOT ONLY THE PRODUCT OF CULTURE. IT
IS STILL, ABOVE ALL, A WORK OF NATURE. WE CAN
ONLY ALTER SO MUCH OF IT ON OUR OWN. BUT WE
CANNOT ESCAPE THE FUNDAMENTAL LAW OF NATURE
THAT EVERYTHING THAT IS NOT USED IS LOST.

You may have noticed that there is a contradiction. On
one hand, you must stay active. On the other, we tell you
that the changes that occur in the body invite us to reduce
activity. At this point, the question is: how is it possible
to stay active with dwindling strength?

Fractals in Nature Abound

A fractal is a figure in which the same pattern can be seen at any scale

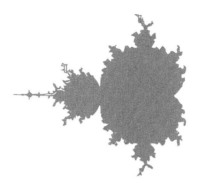

After being discovered by the mathematician Benoît Mandelbrot, it was observed that they are ubiquitous in nature. For example, they are found in:

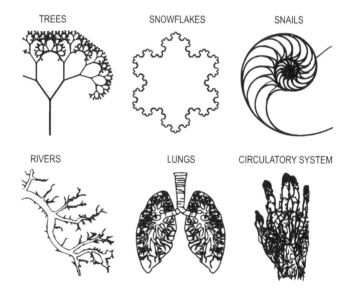

TREES SNOWFLAKES SNAILS

RIVERS LUNGS CIRCULATORY SYSTEM

Source: *The fractal geometry of nature,* by Benoît Mandelbrot

NEVER TOO LATE FOR HEALTHY WORKOUTS

HOW TO MAINTAIN A HEALTHY LEVEL OF PHYSICAL ACTIVITY

We have not yet discussed the metabolism. And yet it is a phenomenon essential to life for its operation and maintenance. The metabolism depends on the function of the cells and tissues of the body—as does longevity, to a large extent.

When we talk about metabolism, we refer to the sum of chemical reactions that take place in the body. For example, the transformation of nutrients into cell components or the accumulation in fat deposits is a metabolic aspect. The transformation of fats into energy is another aspect. On the one side, calories are accumulated, and on the other, calories are burned.

We have all witnessed how metabolism varies from person to person. Some can eat all they want and always remain thin. Others, on the contrary, have a propensity to gain weight even when eating very little.

Why does this injustice occur? Simply because these two types of people do not process the energy from food equally, because their metabolism works differently.

But, unlike many other traits that we cannot alter, such as eye color or the sequence of our genes, our metabolism has the advantage that, to a certain extent, we can regulate it ourselves. Which gives us certain control over our longevity and our quality of life. We can regulate it, especially with physical activity and the food we eat.

> Our metabolism has the advantage that we somewhat regulate it ourselves, especially with the physical activity we do and the food we eat.

As early as the sixteenth century, the Venetian noble Alvise Cornaro wrote an amazing story of survival that, five centuries later, is still enlightening. This is a story that illustrates the relationship between metabolism and longevity. In his *Discourses of a Sober Life*, Cornaro explains how, thanks to his fortune, he enjoyed a life of excess where he gave in to food, drink, and lust. Or rather, half a life of excess. His life of debauchery suddenly came to a halt when, right before turning forty, he felt ill, exhausted, and on the brink of death.

We do not know how sick he was or if his life was in any danger, but it is a mere detail. The point is that his fear of dying led him to change his life. He gave up banquets and orgies. Following the advice of the doctors of his time, he agreed to not eat more than 350 grams of food accompanied by two glasses of wine. He did not follow what we today would call a balanced diet. He ate mostly soup, bread, and egg yolk. But with this diet, which he followed for more than six decades, he lived to be 102. In the times of Cornaro, there was no talk of calories or metabolism. It was not until the last century that science began to take a serious interest in these concepts. And it was not until this last decade that we began to unravel how our metabolism is associated to longevity.

It has been discovered, for example, that the molecule mTOR regulates the growth and metabolism of the body. And when you disable this molecule, it lengthens life in worms, flies, and maybe also in people.

Or that the molecule AMPK, which regulates the consumption of energy by cells, has the opposite effect, as explained in the chart in chapter 19. If mTOR reduces longevity, AMPK increases it. So, activating AMPK (instead of inhibiting it, as with mTOR) lengthens life in mice and—again—maybe also in people.

Another example is the IGF-1 molecule, which we introduced in chapter 3 when we said that it is necessary for growth during childhood and accelerates aging in adulthood. It is another important metabolism regulator and has a similar effect to mTOR: limited longevity.

All these molecules—plus some others—are pieces of an incomplete puzzle. In other areas of research, such as cardiovascular disease or cancer, we have a global theory, and each new discovery helps us to have a more detailed view. In the science of aging, we have many details, but we still lack a complete theory.

However, out of these seemingly unrelated details, an overview is starting to emerge. When one stops to examine what the different interventions that seem to extend life—such as inhibiting mTOR or activator AMPK, among others—have in common, a recurrent pattern emerges: they all force the body to act as if resources were scarce and it had to take advantage of them with maximum efficiency.

This is what experiments indicate. When animals like laboratory mice, flies, and worms are subjected to caloric restriction—a dietary regimen that reduces calorie intake—their metabolism adapts by dedicating available resources to activities essential to the maintenance and repair of the body, while allocating fewer resources to nonessential activities such as regeneration of the tissues, rapid multiplication of the cells, or accumulation of reserves in the form of fat.

This adaptation is done by regulating the molecules that we have discussed, such as inhibiting mTOR and activator AMPK. This is what might have happened to Alvise Cornaro when he gave up his life of excesses. In the case of laboratory animals, the increase of longevity observed in experiments of caloric restriction is amazing. In mice, for example, which are mammals like us and resemble us more than flies or worms do, the median survival has increased by 65 percent, and maximum survival by 50 percent. If these results can be transferred to people one day—which we do not know whether it will happen or not—the average survival would go from about 80 to 100, and maximum survival from 120 to 180. Would any of you like to live that many years?

We have previously mentioned that physical activity is the opposite of diet. If through our diet we accumulate nutrients and calories, physical activity leads us to spend them. It is not surprising, therefore, that the constant practice of physical activity, as well as a calorie-restricted diet, modulates the metabolism and influences longevity.

This effect is evident if you think about what happens at

the level of organs and tissues. Physical activity exercises the cardiorespiratory system and helps keep the heart and lungs in shape. It requires an effort from the muscles, which stay invigorated instead of atrophied. The bones, which respond to the actions of the muscles, stay sturdy, which reduces the risk of fractures in the future.

Even the brain stays in shape with physical activity. When we exercise our coordination and balance, one of the things most affected by age, it helps us stay more agile and more certain of our movements—remember the test in chapter 6. In addition, exercise enhances our ability to concentrate and plan activities, helps preserve memory and spatial orientation, reduces the risk of developing Alzheimer's, and provides a psychological wellbeing that allows us to conserve a good quality of life. If we look at what happens at a microscopic scale, the effect of physical activity is the opposite of excessive dieting. It is particularly important what happens in the muscles, which are the tissues we demand the most from during exercise. Thus, physical activity activates the AMPK molecule, which as we have seen, regulates the metabolism and promotes longevity. It also potentiates the activity of SIRT1 (found in chapter 3), of FOXO3 (chapters 7 and 9), and other molecules with hieroglyphic-looking names.

All these molecules teach the same lesson. Muscles—far from being the passive tissues that merely provide the necessary force to move the body, humble workers that follow the orders of the Great Chief Brain—are, in fact, a true endocrine organ that secretes dozens of molecules essential for the proper functioning of the body. Without our brain, we would not be able to move a muscle. But without muscles, neither the brain nor the body would be able to do much. It takes true teamwork to ensure health and promote longevity. That is why muscle activity is so necessary to enjoying a long existence with a good quality of life.

Of course, physical activity provides many benefits beyond the muscles. If we look at how it affects the blood, it raises the levels of good cholesterol (HDL cholesterol) and reduces bad cholesterol (or LDL). It promotes the activity of insulin, which reduces the risk of developing diabetes. It helps control blood pressure, which prevents or reduces hypertension. And, if we look at the white blood cells, we discover that physical activity helps maintain long telomeres.

You may remember the telomeres from chapter 3. These are structures at the end of the chromosomes that get shorter with age and that we compared to the plastic bits that protect your shoelaces. When comparing the cells of physically active people with sedentary people, the former have longer telomeres. This means that their cells lack a greater number of cell divisions before entering a state of senescence. It also means that there is still life ahead of them. It is further evidence that physical activity has an anti-aging effect.

It also has a psychological effect that indirectly affects longevity and quality of life, which is equally important. People who begin physical activity after years of a sedentary lifestyle begin to take care of other aspects of their health.

The opposite does not usually occur. One can start a diet for weight control, but if it is not coupled with any type of physical activity, chances are that the diet will be abandoned sooner or later. But when one begins to be physically active and finds the time to do it, one becomes conscious of how important it is, because time is our most limited resource. And if you also discover that you enjoy being physically active, that it brings you psychological wellbeing, you probably will persist. As a result, your general state of health and wellbeing will improve.

That's why physical activity is usually the best gateway to healthcare, because it is accompanied by a process of awareness that facilitates accepting responsibility for our own body. It leaves behind the attitude of "Doctor, can you tell me what diet I should follow or pill I should take?" and replaces it with "Doctor, I will take care of it myself."

Physical activity also has another advantage. Its beneficial effects are not confined to the period in which we exercise; they continue for a while afterwards. This is something that everyone who practices physical activity regularly experiences.

That's why physical activity is usually the best gateway to healthcare. Because it is accompanied by an awareness process that facilitates one being responsible for one's own body.

We not only feel better during exercise, but especially in the following hours and even days.

If you exercise only sporadically, you may disagree, because the fatigue may bother you, and the next day you feel exhausted and stiff. But if the physical activity in your life is habitual, you will see how every day you are less tired, every day you enjoy it more, and every day you feel better. A fact that may convince you: sedentary people are more vulnerable to stress and have twice the risk of depressive symptoms than physically active people.

The prolonged benefit of exercise is not only psychological but also metabolic. Active people not only burn more calories than sedentary people when they exercise, but throughout the day as well. Of all the calories spent because of physical activity, approximately half are spent during exercise and the other half in moments of rest.

The explanation is that the body is reprogrammed to burn calories more efficiently.

In the muscles, physical activity augments the number of mitochondria in the cells. Mitochondria are microscopic energy centers, so the more mitochondria a cell has, the more energy it produces and the more calories it burns.

SO, ACTIVE PEOPLE NOT ONLY BURN MORE CALORIES THAN SEDENTARY PEOPLE DO WHILE EXERCISING, BUT THROUGHOUT THE DAY AS WELL. OF ALL THE CALORIES THAT ARE SPENT THROUGH PHYSICAL ACTIVITY, APPROXIMATELY HALF ARE LOST DURING EXERCISE AND THE OTHER HALF IN MOMENTS OF REST. THE EXPLANATION IS THAT THE BODY IS REPROGRAMMED TO BURN CALORIES MORE EFFICIENTLY.

At this point, practical questions may arise. If we want to practice physical activity not only for fun but with our health in mind and to delay the aging process, what is the best choice? How often should we practice it? With what intensity and for how long? And, if we have surrendered to a sedentary lifestyle for years—or to excess, as Alvise Cornaro did—where do we start? Are there any special precautions we should take?

The first recommendation is common sense. You cannot

become addicted to something you do not like. You can try saying to yourself, "I have to do it," but if you do not like it, sooner or later you will drop it. Therefore, seek an activity that you could potentially enjoy. If you have vertigo, do not climb. And if you do not like water, do not swim, even if someone tells you that it is the best thing for you. If you do not like it, it is best to not do it. With the number of different options available, there are some you will probably find more appropriate. Another recommendation is common sense: do not confuse activity with physical sports. Walking is an excellent physical activity, especially a brisk walk, even if it is not a sport. Taking the stairs instead of the elevator is another physical activity. Even gardening, washing the car, or hanging clothes to dry can be a physical activity. The sum of all these small activities, if incorporated in our daily routines, can be better for our health than playing tennis or soccer once a week, or succumbing to a sedentary lifestyle the rest of the week.

If walking and climbing stairs seems like very little and you want more, you should consider that there are different types of physical activity. They are all beneficial and convenient when done correctly. But they are complementary, so it is advisable to combine them. On one hand, we have aerobic activities, in which the muscles need a lot of oxygen for an extended period. To supply them with oxygen, we are forced to breathe faster and deeper, and the heart must beat faster. They are, therefore, ideal activities to exercise the cardiorespiratory system. They are also suitable for increasing physical endurance and burning calories. Racing, which is a classic example of aerobic exercise, is the physical activity that burns the most calories. That is why runners tend to be thinner while swimmers or soccer players have a more robust silhouette.

On the other hand, we have resistance exercises, in which the muscles must overcome opposition. They are ideal to strengthen muscles and bones, and for muscles to segregate all those molecules that favor longevity—previously cited as AMPK, SIRT1, or FOXO3. Classic examples of resistance activities include weights, push-ups, or sit-ups.

But in fact, all physical activity has a cardiorespiratory component and a muscular component. In cycling, for example, the aerobic component predominates on flat areas and resistance when going uphill. In swimming, equally important are the water resistance that must be overcome and the need to keep the muscles well oxygenated so as not to run out of breath. Any of these activities are appropriate if you enjoy them.

Activities with a proprioceptive component, such as dance or tai chi, facilitate control of body movements and, especially in older people, reduce the risk of falls. The only thing that is not recommended, if we enjoy taking care of ourselves and having long-term good health, is to surrender to a sedentary lifestyle.

Once we have decided what physical activity we prefer, all we need is to determine what frequency, duration, and intensity are good for us. It is common to make the mistake of thinking that if something is good, the more we do it, the better. But with the human body, this does not apply. If you remember the concept of homeostasis that we discussed in chapter 5, biological systems work well when they are in a state of balance, not of excess. There is nothing in biology that follows the law of "the more, the better." There always comes a point in which something that was good before is not so good now. And if that continues to happen, you will get to a point where something that was beneficial becomes harmful. It is something that is often observed among people who exercise and go too far and end up hurting themselves due to too much activity.

The million-dollar question is: at what point does "the more, the better" become "the more, the worse"? This point varies depending on the person. Let's look at the average population, as was done in the UK with the Million Women Study, for which healthy women from the ages of fifty to sixty-four were recruited. The women who did some form of physical activity every day had a higher risk of heart attack or stroke than those who exercised every day. And those who did vigorous physical activity had a higher risk than those who were moderately active. Therefore, at least within that age group, the healthiest rate is moderate physical activity three to five times per week.

This result is in line with the recommendations for the general population given by the American Heart Association (AHA), which recommends combining aerobic physical activity with resistance. For aerobic exercise, choose between a moderate activity such as walking at a fast pace (at least thirty minutes per day and at least five days a week) or an intense activity such as running (at least three days a week and at least twenty-five minutes per session). For a resistance activity, they propose bodybuilding exercises at least twice a week, without specifying how long.

In case you want to exercise with machines in the gym, of which there are an astonishing variety, look for those that are more adequate to the type of activity that is convenient for you. If you have questions, ask them and be open to taking advice. For older people, the stationary bike is usually desirable because you do not fall even if you have balance problems, and the pace can be controlled. With the treadmill, however, you must go at the pace set by the machine, and sometimes accidents will happen. One last warning before you lace up your sneakers and go off to play sports: if up until now you have been a member of the Couch Potato Club, do not begin abruptly. Trying to do too much the first few days is the fastest way to an injury. Do not attempt to beat any records from the start. Begin slowly, with moderate intensity, not excessively long efforts, and you can give yourself more demanding challenges in the future.

If it has been years since you did any form of structured exercise, consulting a general practitioner or sports physician before beginning is not a bad idea. They might recommend a stress test to assess if your heart is in good condition for intense physical activity. And the stress test will probably go well, as it generally does. But there are cases of people who suffer a heart attack while doing rigorous physical activity that they were not prepared for. It is always better to have a checkup before starting than to regret not having one.

AEROBIC ACTIVITY

Moderate activity at least 30 minutes, 5 days a week   OR   **Vigorous activity for at least 25 minutes, 3 days a week**

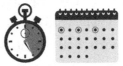

Examples: Examples:

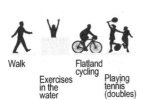

Walk

Exercises
in the
water

Flatland
cycling

Playing
tennis
(doubles)

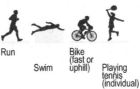

Run

Swim

Bike
(fast or
uphill)

Playing
tennis
(individual)

+

MUSCLE-BUILDING ACTIVITY

Activity at least 2 times a week

Exercises that use all major muscle groups

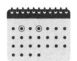

Examples:

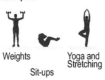

Weights

Sit-ups

Yoga and
Stretching

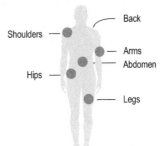

Shoulders

Hips

Back

Arms

Abdomen

Legs

Source: The Centers for Disease Control and Prevention

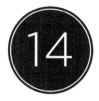

BRAIN FITNESS

THE MYTHS OF COGNITIVE DECLINE

Not everything in the body changes for the worse with age. We have internalized that the aging process is synonymous with decline to such a degree that we do not even realize that some skills tend to improve. You can test this yourself. Ask ten or twenty people what their favorite food is and see how many people will reply that their mother's or grandmother's cooking is their favorite. Do you think that people cooked better one or two generations ago? Of course not. This is the age of Master Chef. It is because intelligence in the kitchen, along with other cognitive skills based on experience, improves with age.

A few decades ago, psychologists realized it was a mistake to look at intelligence as a skill that reaches its peak in youth, then declines slowly but inexorably. This theory is too simple; the human brain is a lot more complex. This was eventually resolved when the notion of two different types of intelligence was introduced.

On one hand, we have fluid intelligence, which reflects the speed at which the brain processes information and is at its peak during early adulthood. On the other hand, there is crystallized intelligence, which is based on the accumulation of experiences and, therefore, continues to develop throughout life.

This distinction explains why grandmothers cook so well or why Gauguin painted his best work during his mature years.

Seen this way, the expert brain works like an old computer that contains a lot of information that it processes very slowly. It is not fast, but it is reliable. That is why those who can give better advice are often older. People who know more than us and have slower reflexes but more wisdom. The voice of experience.

This metaphor of an old computer is mostly correct, but it's incomplete. It is still too simple, because both fluid intelligence and crystallized intelligence encompass different types of skills. And if we examine every aptitude separately, as researchers from Harvard University and Massachusetts General Hospital have done, we see that they do not all evolve equally over a lifetime. In a study where data collected from more than a thousand people was analyzed, it was observed that not all fluid intelligence reaches its maximum potential during our twenties, and not all crystallized intelligence increases progressively. What happens is that at each age, we improve some aspects and others get worse. Therefore, there is no optimal age for intellectual performance. It depends on what concrete aspect of intelligence we value.

In visual search tests, for example, where an object or a face must be found in a multi-colored image, or a product must be found in a store, or the keys when we forget where we left them, the best results are obtained at the end of adolescence. But if you ask us to remember lists of numbers, such as a phone number we forget to write down, our memory will be best equipped for this five years later, between the ages of twenty and twenty-five. If, instead of numbers, we are challenged to memorize a list of words and then repeat them backwards, we will be best at this between the ages of thirty and thirty-five.

All these are examples of fluid intelligence, in which the brain must process information in the short term without having to store it as memory. As you can see, each part matures at its own pace.

If, however, we test our crystallized intelligence, for example in vocabulary games, defining words, or games of general knowledge like Trivial Pursuit, we will obtain the best results around the age of fifty.

But the most interesting result to come from the study by Harvard University and Massachusetts General Hospital is probably the test in which participants were asked to recognize emotions in the eyes of other people. It is not an easy test. A computer screen displays the eyes of various people and prompts the participant to choose from a menu that includes options such as "indecision," "bewilderment," "surprise," or "skepticism."

This skill is useful when working in a team, dealing with strangers, communicating with our spouse or children, or navigating the world in general. It is a fundamental part of emotional intelligence. At what age would you say it reaches its peak? It is not as early as the components of fluid intelligence or as late as the components of crystallized intelligence. The best time to interpret someone else's emotions is, on average, between the age of forty and sixty.

All this demonstrates that the brain, like any other organ, changes with age. But this change does not have to be seen as a progressive and irremediable loss of powers. Rather, as the years pass, something is lost and something is gained.

These changes in the functioning of the brain are reflected in its anatomy. The same way the muscles lose strength or skin becomes thinner with age, the brain also loses mass and volume. About 25 percent for people between the ages of thirty and eighty, according to a study that evaluated the brains of people of different ages using magnetic resonance imaging.

Much of this loss is concentrated in the final years, during the same period in which other organs atrophy. The loss is not uniform throughout the brain. It is more pronounced in the white matter, which is formed primarily by neural wiring (or axons) that connect the different regions of the brain, which in the gray matter, is formed by the central body of the neurons.

Even in gray matter, researchers have observed a loss of 14 percent in the frontal lobe, which regulates important functions such as planning and decision-making abilities, moral behavior or voluntary control of movement. Another observation was a 13 percent loss in the hippocampus, which controls memory and spatial orientation and is one of the brain structures most affected by Alzheimer's disease.

This certainly does not sound like good news. If we look at what happens at a microscopic level, the results are not much more encouraging. The myelin, which is the substance that wraps around the wiring of the neurons, like the plastic tubes that line electrical wires, degrades, causing the transmission of nerve impulses to become less efficient. The connection between neurons (or synapse) becomes less dense. And, within the synapses, some important neurotransmitters (which are molecules that transmit information from one neuron to another) become scarcer.

This is what happens, for example, with dopamine, a neurotransmitter that acts as a conductor and controls multiple functions—from the movements of the body to motivation, from attention to sleep. Or with the glutamate, the main excitatory neurotransmitter used by the brain. Or with serotonin, which regulates emotional wellness.

But do not be discouraged. Nothing is more capable than the brain at adapting to changes. Unlike other organs, the brain is in permanent renewal to perceive how the world around it changes, to learn new tasks, to continue acquiring memories and generating original ideas.

You can learn a new language or how to play an instrument at any age. Some thousands of neurons reorganize their connections so that we internalize how we must coordinate our movements to go from a C to Dm or how to say good morning in German. This is what is referred to as neuroplasticity.

No organ is more capable than the brain at adapting to changes. Unlike other organs, the brain is in constant renewal to perceive how the world changes around it, to learn new tasks, and to continue acquiring memories and generating original ideas.

Alright, it is more difficult to learn German or to play the guitar at the age of seventy-five than at fifteen, and if we got a late start, we will hardly become a guitar virtuoso. But the capacity for learning is not lost. The cognitive functions of the brain are like heartbeats. They remain until death. What happens is that the more data we have accumulated in the past, the more crystallized intelligence we have acquired, the harder it is to introduce new data into the system. Like our old computer, our memory is full.

YOU CAN LEARN A NEW LANGUAGE OR A MUSICAL INSTRUMENT TO PLAY AT ANY AGE. SOME THOUSANDS OF NEURONS REORGANIZE THEIR CONNECTIONS AND INTERNALIZE HOW TO COORDINATE MOVEMENTS FROM C TO DM OR HOW TO SAY GOOD MORNING IN GERMAN. IT IS CALLED NEURAL PLASTICITY.

When we have reached this point, it is natural to ask ourselves if there is anything we can do to keep the brain in shape. To do a memory expansion, so to speak, such as something like the aerobic exercises for the cardiorespiratory system explained in the previous chapter, or the resistance exercises for muscles, but designed specifically for the brain. The answer is yes. There are two types of activities that have proven to be useful in preventing cognitive decline. On one side, intellectual activities. On the other, physical activities.

Let us begin with the intellectual activities. You may have already heard that doing Sudoku or crossword puzzles is good for maintaining mental agility. If only that were true. Unfortunately, there is no data to support it. It is not necessarily bad. If you like doing Sudoku puzzles, do not stop now.

But it is not clear that doing Sudoku puzzles instructs the brain to do anything except more Sudokus. It is different than learning to play a musical instrument, which requires attention, concentration, and coordination, as well as an intuitive knowledge of the relationship between the notes. It is definitely a general mobilization of intelligence, and it improves other skills as well. In fact, there are multiple studies that indicate that studying music helps improve attention span, intelligence, and academic performance in children and adolescents. And some studies suggest that playing a musical instrument in adulthood protects against cognitive decline years later.

Speaking different languages also has a protective effect

on the brain. Bilingual people with Alzheimer's often develop the first symptoms of the disease four to five years later than those who speak only one language. Which means that speaking several languages provides the brain with a cognitive reserve, a margin of safety, to continue to function well in adverse conditions. It is like a car that embarks on a difficult journey with a good reserve of fuel in the tank. The more reserve it has, the further it will get before problems arise.

What, then, do music and languages have that Sudoku puzzles and crossword puzzles do not? Possibly that they enhance neuroplasticity. This is a nascent field of research, and we still have more questions than answers. But the most beneficial activities seem to be those that require an effort to learn.

When we demand that the brain do something a little more difficult than what it normally does comfortably—when we make it step out of its comfort zone—it adapts by reorganizing part of its neurons so that the next time it is easier. Conversely, when we offer the brain a more contemplative practice that is also an intellectual activity, such as watching a movie or doing a hobby, it has no need to adapt. If you stop and think about it, it is not surprising. The same happens when we exercise our muscles or the cardiorespiratory system. We only improve our performance when we demand a little more than what is comfortable.

Unfortunately, little is known of what specific intellectual activities are more useful in preventing cognitive decline. What is good for the brain—to cook? Read or write? Listen to Mozart? Do mental calculations? Read the newspaper and stay informed? Travel? The truth is that no one knows exactly. The most that we can do for now is to propose a hypothesis: probably any of these activities can prevent cognitive decline, but it depends on the attitude with which we do them. Cooking creatively will help you more than just following a recipe. If you do mental calculations in a way that is a little harder for you, it will also be more useful than doing them the straightforward way. If you use maps to find your way when you travel, you will retain your sense of direction better than if you are always guided by the GPS.

Further research regarding the relationship between physical activity and cognitive performance has been conducted. Here, the data is unequivocal. At any age, from infancy to old age, the practice of physical activity improves the functioning of the brain. In school, physically active children on average outperform sedentary children on tests of perception, memory, intelligence, and verbal and math skills.

In adults, cardiorespiratory fitness has been associated with improved intellectual performance. In older people, cognitive capabilities improve, or at least do not diminish, with physical activity.

Much of this effect is explained due to the lack of aerobic physical activity associated with insufficient blood flow to the brain. A well-oxygenated, well-fed brain will work better than one that suffers from suffocation. Just like any other organ, it is less efficient when deprived of blood.

In adults, cardiorespiratory fitness has been associated with improved intellectual performance. In older people, cognitive capabilities improve, or at least do not diminish, with physical activity.

In the absence of physical activity, the blood vessels of the brain tend to degrade, which slowly but irreversibly causes extensive damage to the brain. It has been observed that a person with good cardiovascular fitness has lower risk of cognitive decline in old age.

Conversely, the idea that Alzheimer's and cardiovascular diseases are independent is incorrect. Today, we know that a flow of poor blood circulation to the brain exacerbates Alzheimer's.

Resistance exercises, which work out the muscles more than the cardiorespiratory system, have also proven to be beneficial to the brain. If it seems implausible, remember that the muscles act as organs that secrete substances throughout the body.

An informative study from King's College London may

convince you. Three hundred twenty-four pairs of twins participated, with an average age of fifty-five at the beginning of the study. They were given a muscle strength and a neuropsychological test; each pair was tested to assess who was stronger and what their cognitive abilities were. Would you guess what was observed ten years later? Those with more muscular strength showed little decline in intellectual performance. They had what could be called, without exaggeration, mental strength. It was also observed, using a neuroimaging technique, that the weaker the musculature of a person, the more the brain had changed and lost volume.

This does not mean that we must dedicate ourselves to bodybuilding. Apply common sense. There is a level of muscular development that will not provide additional benefits, and an excess of muscles can be just as damaging as a deficit, if not more. What the King's College London study indicates is that a certain level of muscle activity is necessary for the good of the body and we should not ignore it.

Even coordination activities—in which the proprioceptive component predominates and improves the control of body movements—are beneficial to the functioning of the brain. It has been observed, for example, that learning a new motor activity induces the formation of specialized cells in the brain. These cells are responsible for the production of myelin, the substance that covers the wiring of neurons and that is lost with age. Therefore, exercises that require good coordination of movement may be helpful in limiting the loss of myelin and maintaining good neuronal activity.

Together, all these studies point in the same direction. They indicate that all types of physical activity are beneficial, and that they are so for multiple structures and functions of the nervous system. They are beneficial for blood flow; for the connections between neurons; for limiting the loss of brain volume; for the hippocampus, which is a key region in memory and spatial orientation; for the prefrontal cortex, which is key to planning and making decisions...They are pretty much good for almost the entire brain.

So do not give up. Cognitive faculties change with age; it is inevitable. We might lose certain skills, but in exchange, we acquire new ones. We can live this process as a decline or we can live it as an adaptation. It is largely up to us, because there is so much we can do to keep our brain in shape. And it is not that the passage of time is not important. Of course it is. But age is not the only variable on which the cognitive state depends in healthy people. There is another equally important variable: attitude.

Functional anatomy of the brain...

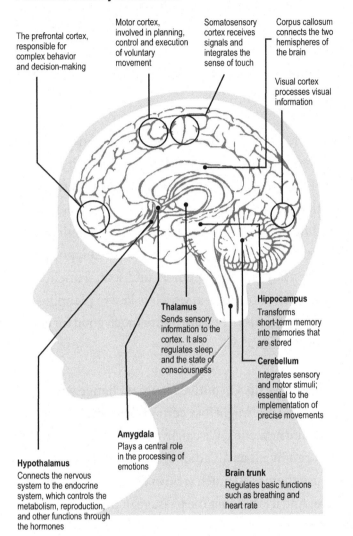

The prefrontal cortex, responsible for complex behavior and decision-making

Motor cortex, involved in planning, control and execution of voluntary movement

Somatosensory cortex receives signals and integrates the sense of touch

Corpus callosum connects the two hemispheres of the brain

Visual cortex processes visual information

Thalamus
Sends sensory information to the cortex. It also regulates sleep and the state of consciousness

Hippocampus
Transforms short-term memory into memories that are stored

Cerebellum
Integrates sensory and motor stimuli; essential to the implementation of precise movements

Amygdala
Plays a central role in the processing of emotions

Hypothalamus
Connects the nervous system to the endocrine system, which controls the metabolism, reproduction, and other functions through the hormones

Brain trunk
Regulates basic functions such as breathing and heart rate

...and of a neuron

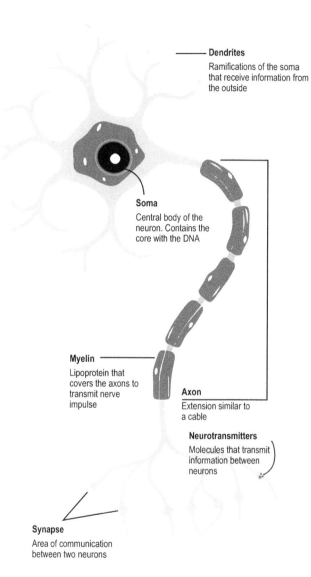

Dendrites
Ramifications of the soma that receive information from the outside

Soma
Central body of the neuron. Contains the core with the DNA

Myelin
Lipoprotein that covers the axons to transmit nerve impulse

Axon
Extension similar to a cable

Neurotransmitters
Molecules that transmit information between neurons

Synapse
Area of communication between two neurons

KEEP ON SMILING

THERE'S NO PHYSICAL WELLBEING WITHOUT EMOTIONAL WELLBEING

Remember Jeanne Calment, the woman who lived to be 122 years old that we introduced you to in the chapter about centenarians? You may recall her joking her name was Calment because of how calm she was. She exaggerated, of course. Her calmness was not the reason behind her name. But it was possibly the reason behind her longevity.

It will be no surprise to you if we say that anxiety and stress, which are the opposite of calm and serenity, accelerate aging and shorten our life. It is something that we might have observed in the people around us—perhaps it has even happened to us.

As in the case, for example, of those who appear to have

aged several years in just a few weeks during a serious personal or family crisis. When we see them again after some time, they look beaten, perhaps grayer or with more wrinkles, and when we look into their eyes, they seem older and wiser.

It is also the case for those with sick relatives, such as parents with dementia or children with a serious illness, and who bear the additional burden of stress related to overwork, lack of time for themselves, and the emotional cost of seeing their loved ones suffer.

The changes in the skin and eyes experienced by these people who are subjected to high levels of stress are not anecdotal or superficial. They reflect the deep damage, some of it irreversible, that occurs in the intimacy of the cells. A person's physical appearance corresponds quite accurately with their biological age, as shown by the research conducted by Duke University, explained in chapter 1. Thus, this appearance of accelerated aging caused by stress corresponds with rapid biological aging.

It should be clarified, before proposing antidotes and solutions, that not everything caused by stress is damaging. Stress reactions are, in origin, a basic mechanism of survival in animals that tell the body to fight or flee. Stress is what allows them to react to threats. It allows giraffes to escape lions and people to stay out of the way of a snake or a moving truck.

Precisely because it activates the body, a certain level of stress is healthy, convenient, and even pleasant. There is stress in riding a roller coaster, playing an important final match, preparing for a trip, or working in the E.R. The problem comes when these moderate and functional levels of stress soar, and what was originally a beneficial reaction becomes detrimental.

It should also be clarified that there are different types of harmful stress that affect our health differently. We have, at one extreme, episodes of acute, explosive stress, in which the adrenal glands—located at the top of each kidney—release a burst of cortisol and adrenaline, and we lose total control of the situation. This is what happens, for example, in a fit of anger or a panic attack. For a healthy person, these reactions are harmless to his or her health, although they can certainly be unpleasant for that person and for those around him or her. However, for a person with a poor cardiovascular health, episodes of acute stress are high-risk situations, since the adrenaline can provoke tachycardia, arrhythmias, and sudden increase in blood pressure, which can trigger a cardiac arrest or a stroke.

A CERTAIN LEVEL OF STRESS IS HEALTHY, CONVENIENT, AND PLEASANT BECAUSE IT ACTIVATES THE BODY. THERE IS STRESS IN RIDING A ROLLER COASTER, PLAYING AN IMPORTANT FINAL MATCH, PREPARING FOR A TRIP, OR WORKING IN THE E.R. THE PROBLEM COMES WHEN THESE STRESS LEVELS SOAR AND WHAT WAS A BENEFICIAL REACTION BECOMES DAMAGING.

At the other extreme, we have a less visible type of stress, but it is more insidious and more damaging long term. It is chronic stress. We can learn to live with it, adapt to it, and in the end, accept it as normal, but it will gradually undermine our emotional wellbeing and quality of life. This is the type of stress that caregivers or sick people experience.

Researcher Elizabeth Blackburn, who received the Nobel Prize in Medicine for the discovery of telomeres, has studied the effects of this type of chronic stress on longevity. Telomeres, again, are the DNA sequences that protect the ends of the chromosomes and shorten with age. Blackburn, along with other researchers, compared telomere length between two groups of women. They all had children and were relatively young and healthy. They were an average age of thirty-eight years old. The main difference between the two groups was that, in one, the mothers were responsible for caring for a child with a chronic illness and, in the other, the children were healthy. The women were asked how long they had cared for their children and were surveyed to evaluate their subjective perception of stress.

The results show that the more years they had been caring for their sick child, the more years of accumulated stress, the shorter the telomeres and the less amount of telomerase, the enzyme that is in charge of preserving the telomeres. And the more oxidative activity detected in the cells, which is another damaging process.

When analyzing the results of the survey, the influence of stress was confirmed. The more overwhelmed the mothers felt, both the mothers with the sick children and the ones with healthy children, the shorter the telomeres. Therefore, presumably, they had aged further.

Tests were conducted to see whether this could be the result of smoking. Maybe the women who experienced more stress smoked more and that had shortened the telomeres. But, once the research concluded, the idea was discarded. It was not the tobacco.

They tested once again to see if it could be related to diet. Maybe the women who were more stressed ate worse. But it was not the diet either. It was even thought that maybe it could be related to the use of oral contraceptives. In the end, the only variable that explained the shortening of the telomeres and premature aging was stress. And its effects were daunting.

The researchers compared the 25 percent of women who suffered more stress with the 25 percent who were less stressed. They observed that the stress of caring for a sick child caused premature aging, estimated on the length of the telomeres, of ten years on average.

But that is not everything. The telomeres are one of the targets of stress that affect longevity, but not the only one. There are other more important targets. For example, the immune system and, more specifically, how it regulates inflammation reactions.

Inflammation is primarily a defense mechanism. In the face of aggression or accidental damage—be it a virus, the sting of a scorpion, or a shock—the immune system mobilizes an army of cells to repel the enemy and protect us. These are the cells responsible for the redness, swelling, and increased temperature in the affected area. Even from a fever in case of an infection such as the flu. They are also greatly responsible for the discomfort and pain we experience. A disproportionate inflammatory reaction, although initially intended to help us, results in the opposite effect. And a more moderate but persistent inflammatory activity also becomes a harmful situation that, far from protecting us, causes damage and accelerated aging.

The medical world has coined the term inflammaging. It is a blend of the words inflammation and aging, and it shows how important the role of inflammation is in premature aging.

What happens in situations of chronic stress is that they come with states of chronic inflammation. This phenomenon of chronic stress has been observed in people who feel alone, who have become unemployed, who live in poverty, who have been widowed, diagnosed with a cancer...It has been observed in multiple situations and in many studies.

Research has uncovered why it happens. Chronic stress causes a cascade of biochemical reactions that have an impact on the blood stem cells in the bone marrow. The production of blood, therefore, is affected, although not much, fortunately. The bone marrow continues to produce millions of red blood cells and white blood cells every second, which cannot be stopped any more than we can stop breathing. But there is a type of cell whose production increases in situations of chronic stress: monocytes, the cells that cause inflammation.

Therefore, the sequence of cause and effect, in a nutshell, is as follows: chronic stress increases the production of monocytes, the monocytes cause inflammation, and inflammation can cause premature aging.

So, if we want to get to the root of the problem, to prevent premature aging we must combat chronic stress. For those who suffer from stress, this may seem like an impossible mission.

I can hear you saying, "I would sure love to, doctor, but given the life I have, I am not sure how I can do that." It is understandable, with the life you lead, but do not despair. Remember the U of happiness that we explained in chapter 10? Nearly everyone, with age, learns to live with less stress. And there are two strategies that have proven to be effective in mitigating chronic stress that might be useful.

Stress, if you think about it, is a loss of control over oneself. It occurs in moments of intense stress, such as in the earlier examples of rage or panic. But there is also chronic stress, where each day we go through situations that we do not choose to be in, but we feel controlled by circumstances. The way to beat stress is to not allow our surroundings to control us; in other words, to regain control. This, of course, is easier said than done. One strategy is to become physically active. It might seem like a cure-all, but it has proven to be most effective. Many studies have observed in people of all ages that physical activity is associated with greater emotional wellbeing.

The causal relationship goes both ways. People tend to be more active when they feel well. But they also feel better when they are more active. It has been demonstrated in a type of study called intervention, in which a group of volunteers is asked to perform a certain type of activity which is then compared with another group of volunteers that do not perform the activity. The results show the habitual practice of a physical activity—such as yoga, tai chi, power-walking, or swimming—improves emotional wellbeing.

From this we can conclude that physical activity is also psychological activity. It is not something we are aware of, but to exercise regularly, we must first find the time and then organize our time to do it. Therefore, we must regain a certain control over our schedule. We will decide that from two to three in the afternoon, for example, we will not accept a work meeting but instead will go to the gym or pool. This is a good start to reducing stress.

Physical activity also provides a feeling of self-confidence, of being able to overcome challenges or difficulties, which is extremely useful when confronting the small daily problems that we all have. When one has cycled to the Alpe d'Huez or climbed the Aneto or committed to run ten kilometers in less than forty-five minutes and achieved it, whatever the goal, this helps reassess difficulties that may come up. When Monday rolls around and we must go back to work, we must not let ourselves be dragged by the tide of demands and stress.

In the specific case of yoga, it provides an additional benefit that goes beyond a strictly physical aspect. By emphasizing breathing and meditation, besides mastering posture techniques that allow a sense of control over the body, yoga helps combat stress and promotes emotional balance. In some hospitals today, it is recommended that patients recovering from a heart attack practice yoga.

We said that there are two effective strategies to mitigate chronic stress and that the first is physical activity. The second one is social activity. If you remember the chapter about the blue zones and the people with the highest life expectancy in the world, a point common to all of them was the importance of social relations. In the Greek island of Ikaria and the Barbagia region of Sardinia, family and community are fundamental values. The Seventh-day Adventists of Loma Linda, California, maintain close ties with each other and devote Saturdays to church activities. In the Japanese island of Okinawa, we discussed the case of the 103-year-old woman who spent many hours every day having tea and talking with childhood friends.

In these apparent coincidences, there are no accidents. What we have are causalities with the most advanced U. It is easy to understand why. Humans are social animals, and we need to communicate. Just like the orca in captivity who, separated from other orcas, is unhappy and develops behavioral disorders, an isolated individual goes into decline. It is a very basic biological need, common among social mammals.

The details vary depending on the person. Some feel comfortable in large meetings and others are better in small groups. There are those who are more open with others and those who are more introverted. Those who know how to establish a good relationship with a dog or a horse. And the ones who retire to a hermitage to communicate with God or with nature. Or the ones who look up at the sky at night, looking for signs of alien life. Details vary, but the basic principle remains—we all need to relate.

When analyzing the effects of an active social life on emotional wellness, as researchers have done at Missouri's Washington University in St. Louis, studying people over age sixty, the benefits are clear. They studied whether people who contribute to the community through some type of volunteer work—for example, in a church or in an ONG—feel better than those who do not. And they noted that, in both men and women, an average of two hours per week of volunteering leads to a significantly higher sense of emotional wellbeing.

> In both men and women, an average of two hours per week of volunteer work leads to a significantly higher sense of emotional wellbeing.

An earlier study by the University of Michigan found that, among older people that do volunteer work, the mortality rate is similar to that of people doing physical activity, and lower than in the rest of the population. This raised the question of what was cause and what was effect. Do they volunteer because they feel well, or do they feel well because they volunteer?

Other studies that followed a group of people for periods of up to eight years have clarified the question. Although the initial situation of two people might be the same, over the years, the person who does some type of volunteer work feels better, especially if their contribution feels valuable and they feel like others appreciate them.

> If you want to maintain good emotional health, do what you can to help others and to maintain a social life—if not vibrant, at least active.

If you would like to maintain good emotional health, and not just live more years, but also enjoy them, do not isolate yourself. Do what you can to help others and try to maintain a social life—if not vibrant, at least active. It is not always easy, we know. When a person has low self-esteem and does not feel appreciated, or when they are afraid of being an annoyance, or when they feel like they have isolated themselves from the world for so long that they have no one to speak to, sometimes they would rather stay home. But even in these cases, it is worth giving it a shot. There will always be a place that needs your help and will welcome you with open arms.

Stress Damages Long-Term Health

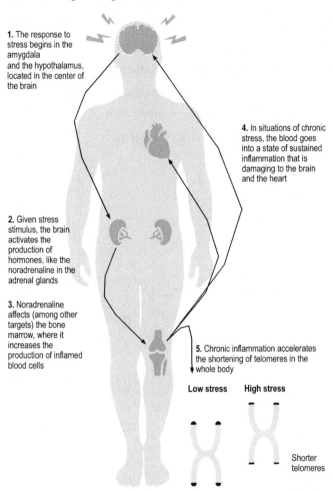

1. The response to stress begins in the amygdala and the hypothalamus, located in the center of the brain

4. In situations of chronic stress, the blood goes into a state of sustained inflammation that is damaging to the brain and the heart

2. Given stress stimulus, the brain activates the production of hormones, like the noradrenaline in the adrenal glands

3. Noradrenaline affects (among other targets) the bone marrow, where it increases the production of inflamed blood cells

5. Chronic inflammation accelerates the shortening of telomeres in the whole body

Low stress   High stress

Shorter telomeres

Source: Nature Medicine/ PNAS

16

SEX HAS NO AGE

HOW TO MAINTAIN AN ACTIVE SEX LIFE DESPITE PREJUDICE AND PHYSIOLOGICAL CHANGES

The same thing that happens with the brain also happens with sex. We are so accustomed to age-related prejudice, we have internalized the concept of decline to such an extent, that we end up accepting as normal that our sex life nears extinction with each new birthday, the same way we accept as normal that intellectual activity decreases. We accept as normal things that are not. They are just prejudices.

Some of you may feel skeptical. "What do these guys know?" you might be thinking. "How can they say there is no decline in sexual activity? They should have seen me at twenty-five—that was activity!" You have a point.

We are not sexually active at twenty-five the way we are at seventy-five. But tennis is not played the same way, either, and yet you still find it normal for a seventy-year-old to play tennis, don't you? A person adapts his way of playing to the circumstances of each moment and can still mark points, games, sets. So why does it seem less normal for a seventy-five-year-old to maintain an active sexual life? Perhaps because, more than *Homo sapiens*, sometimes we are *Homo judgmental*.

The best antidote against prejudice, as we know, is information. It is revealing that there is little data on the sexuality of the elderly. Diet, physical activity, blood pressure, cholesterol, and cognitive skills are studied in detail... why not sex? Not a question we ask of older people, as if it did not exist. But it does exist. And it is an important component of wellbeing. Especially for men, but also for many women. This is what the data says.

> If acceptable health is maintained, sexual interest and ability need not disappear with age.

There are few, but the few that are there convey a clear message: if acceptable health is maintained, sexual interest and ability do not need to disappear with age.

Pioneers of sexology Alfred Kinsey at Indiana University and William Masters and Virginia Johnson at Washington University were the first to study sexuality in older people. They were also the ones who used data to demonstrate that homosexuality is not a disease; that oral sex is a common practice; that some women can have several orgasms, while some men have a refractory period between orgasms; or that masturbation doesn't cause acne, loss of intellectual facilities, or any other disorder. Seen now, it is astounding that only sixty years ago these things were not known. Nothing better than science to dismantle prejudice and discrimination.

The studies of Kinsey and Masters and Johnson, however, were not sufficient to dispel the taboo around sexuality in older people. Although it has been demonstrated that there is no age at which sexual interest and the ability to experience pleasure diminish, today there is still an epidemic of ignorance surrounding this issue.

Masters and Johnson observed that over the years, there are changes in the sexual response of men and women. Men take longer to feel sexually aroused, they may need manual stimulation to get an erection, and when they do, it is not as vigorous as in youth, and ejaculation is not as powerful. Women also take longer to reach a state of arousal, they experience changes in the anatomy of the vagina, which becomes shorter and narrower, and the volume of vaginal lubrication is reduced. These changes are perfectly normal and do not prevent a satisfactory sex life.

In fact, in surveys of sexual satisfaction, women declare themselves to be more satisfied after the age of fifty than before, partly because they no longer need to worry about the possibility of an unwanted pregnancy, which in part gives them greater control over their sexuality. In the National Health and Sexual conduct study done in the United States in 2010, the opposite trend was observed between men and women. While in men the probability of having an orgasm during sex diminishes progressively from the age of eighteen to fifty-nine years old, women experience the opposite effect: the probability of having an orgasm increases over the same age span.

But the most interesting part of the survey, for those interested in the science of long life and reaching advanced ages in full physical and mental health, is what emerges after the age of sixty.

In Spain, in a survey conducted in 2005, 34 percent of people over the age of sixty-five (one in three people) had sexual relations with their partner in the past month. Of these, half had them within the last week. In the United States, according to 2010 data, around 25 percent of men and women (one in four people) remained sexually active after their eightieth birthday.

Consider some detailed data from a study conducted by doctors at the Karolinska hospital in Stockholm on men between the ages of fifty and eighty, who represent half the population of Sweden. The study was limited to men because it stemmed from a larger project on the effects of prostate cancer and the patient's subsequent quality of life.

The results show that 84 percent of men experience sexual desire at least three times a month in the sixth decade of life (between the ages of fifty and fifty-nine). The percentage drops to 49 percent in the seventh decade and 26 percent in the eighth. They observed the same downward trend for the ability to have an erection, the frequency of orgasms (both in couple relations and through masturbation), and for intercourse. Eighty-three percent of men between fifty and fifty-nine reported having sex as a couple at least once a month, 48 percent between sixty and sixty-nine, and 34 percent between the ages of seventy and seventy-nine years old.

But the study was not limited to recording the frequency of sexual activity at different ages. Its great merit is that it asked how men psychologically experienced the decline of sexual function. The conclusion is summarized in one word: bad. When asked how important it was to them to be able to experience sexual desire, to have an erection, and to experience an orgasm, seven out of ten said they considered it relevant to their quality of life past the age of seventy.

Let us take the example of the orgasm. Between the ages

of fifty and fifty-nine, it is important to 96 percent of men, and about 95 percent experience it at least once a month; in this age group, there is no problem. Ten years later, it remains important for 89 percent, but only 75 percent experience it. Here is where it begins to show a discrepancy between what you want and what you can actually have. In those over seventy, the distance widens: it is important for 73 percent of them, but only 46 percent experience it. The same trends, with a growing discrepancy between wanting and doing, have been observed in the other variables analyzed, such as the ability to have an erection, sexual desire, or the volume of ejaculation.

If it is so important to maintain an active sex life, and yet so many people experience a decline, living with frustration or resignation, we should ask ourselves what are the determining factors of a satisfied sex life or lack thereof. This way, we can see what we need to do to maintain a satisfactory degree of sexual activity.

It depends on two key variables, according to the 2010 United States National Health and Sexual Conduct Survey. One is the kind of relationship we have. The other is the state of health.

It is no surprise that people in a relationship have a higher probability of being sexually active at any age. But even among those who have a partner, there is a great variability. When a doctor asks a patient to discuss his personal life, and the patient agrees, which does not always happen, it is not uncommon to find that there is lack of communication between intimate partners. Mutual misunderstanding is a great obstacle, not only to a satisfactory sex life, but also to emotional wellbeing in a broader sense.

One of the most common problems is what sexologists call discrepancy in desire. It means that the frequency of sexual relations between a couple does not correspond with what they actually want. If this has never happened to you, you are an exception. Do you think it is the norm to have a partner whom you want and desire, and for that love and attraction to be reciprocal? And for both to have the same frequency of sexual desire, and that this coincidence will last a lifetime? Maybe this is plausible in fiction—in a novel or in a movie—but it is not what happens in real life. What happens is that, even when a couple is perfectly in sync at the beginning of their relationship, it is inevitable that the desire will evolve over time, and it is common that it will not be synchronized perfectly.

If the relationship is good, this discrepancy in desire does not need to become a serious problem. In fact, many couples adapt to it and find strategies to avoid problems.

If the relationship is damaged and the couple believes that it is normal to stop having sex as they get older, then it will be more difficult to have a satisfactory sex life. Unless they go to couples therapy, they will end up adding to the population group for whom, as in the Swedish study, there is an insurmountable difference between what they want and what they can have.

In addition to these psychological problems that affect sexuality, physiological factors can also interfere. In men, though not serious, it is more common for there to be a progressive decline in testosterone with age, which is associated with a decline in sexual activity, physical performance, muscle mass, and a feeling of vitality. This has led to many men resorting to testosterone supplements, usually without medical supervision, with the hope of not declining. This in turn has led to the U.S. National Institutes of Health to fund clinical trials to assess the effectiveness and risks of testosterone supplements.

At the time of writing this book, the first results of short-term and medium-term efficacy have just been released, and there is a lack of perspective to assess the long-term side effects. The efficacy data show that, in men over the age of sixty-five, testosterone supplements have a positive but moderate effect on sexual desire, erectile function, and sexual activity until up to one year after starting the treatment. They have a positive but also moderate effect on mood, and they do not have a significant effect on feelings of vitality.

It is suspected that testosterone may come with certain risks. Among these, and which have not been proven or ruled out, are potential side effects on the prostate and cardiovascular health.

With the data available to date, the positive effects in men over sixty-five are moderate, the effects in men younger than sixty-five are unknown, and it is not yet known if the potential risks justify the benefits. Therefore, there are not sufficient arguments to recommend testosterone supplements, except in cases in which there is a pathological deficit of the hormone.

An even worse problem than the decline of testosterone to maintain an active sex life, and very common, is poor cardiovascular health. Think about how an erection depends on a complex network of veins and arteries that control the blood irrigation system of the penis. Everything that might harm good circulation of the blood throughout the body also damages the circulation in the genital area and, therefore, a man's erection, as well as the irrigation of the clitoris in women. We must remember that the clitoris is formed during the fetal development of girls from the same tissue that forms the penis in boys, which helps us understand why it is so rich in nerve endings and why it is so important to pleasure. The influence of the blood flow in the genital area explains how the major risk factors for erectile dysfunction are the same ones for cardiovascular diseases: high tension, smoking, obesity, sedentary lifestyle, and the excess of cholesterol. And that the main antidotes are also the same: a healthy diet and an active lifestyle.

If you want specific data, smoking increases the risk of erectile dysfunction by 50 percent, and obesity by more than 90 percent. By contrast, moderate physical activity, equivalent to running thirty minutes three times a week, reduces it by 30 percent, according to a study from the Harvard School of Public Health, led by Eric Rimm and based on data of 22,000 men.

A healthy diet also helps maintain good sexual function. The Mediterranean diet has proven to have a greater protective effect, which is not surprising, given that it has proven to be more suitable for the prevention of cardiovascular diseases.

Within the Mediterranean diet, another study led by Eric Rimm at Harvard has analyzed what foods are more beneficial. The revised data is based on more than 25,000 men who responded every four years to a detailed survey on their lifestyle and health. The survey included a battery of questions about their diet, as well as a few questions about their sexual function.

The results show that the foods rich in flavonoids are the

most helpful in preventing erectile dysfunction. No other similar studies have been conducted to assess which foods promote a satisfactory sex life in women, but it is probably not as important, as the female sexual experience does not depend so much on the blood flow to the genital organs. In any case, to the extent that it depends on the blood flow, there is no reason to think that the beneficial foods would be very different.

FOODS RICH IN FLAVONOIDS ARE THE MOST HELPFUL TO PREVENT ERECTILE DYSFUNCTION. NO SIMILAR STUDIES HAVE BEEN DONE TO KNOW WHICH FOODS FAVOR A SATISFACTORY SEX LIFE IN WOMEN, BUT IT IS PROBABLY NOT AS IMPORTANT, GIVEN THAT THE FEMALE SEXUAL EXPERIENCE DOES NOT DEPEND AS MUCH ON BLOOD FLOW.

If you want to have a diet rich in flavonoids, you should be happy to hear it is not difficult. Flavonoids are a large group of substances of plant origin found in many foods. They abound in berries, citrus fruits, in parsley, in cocoa, in red wine, in tea, in coffee...There is even a study that found that in the US population, drinking two to three cups of coffee a day reduces the risk of erectile dysfunction in 39 percent of men. The explanation is that some flavonoids act on molecules that regulate the subtle balance between the constriction and dilation of the blood vessels of the penis.

Because erection depends on this balance, and because almost all drugs prescribed to patients with cardiovascular diseases affect vasoconstriction and vasodilation, it is not uncommon for these patients to experience a loss of sexual function. These are cases in which the problem does not come from cardiovascular disease, but from the drugs prescribed to treat it.

If doctors do not ask, these patients will not talk about it. They tend to view it with resignation, as something that cannot be changed. They think that there comes a time when people withdraw from sex, like an athlete withdraws from competition. He retires and will never again feel the sweet taste of victory. Besides, what will the doctor even say? That it is not that serious. After all, what importance can an erection have compared to a heart attack? But if a doctor asks them during a medical appointment, it turns out that it is important to them. Very important to many men.

And although there is no guarantee of success, there are strategies for a possible solution. In the case of patients who take multiple drugs, as is usual for people with cardiac diseases, a strategy that tends to work is to stop taking one drug at a time and see what happens, because there are many drugs that can cause sexual dysfunction in predisposed patients.

Doctors can start by removing beta blockers for blood pressure, because those act on the beta receptors that regulate vasodilation. Therefore, it is a type of drug that directly affects the mechanism of erection. If no improvement is observed after two weeks, the patient can resume taking the beta blockers. Next they can stop taking the drug for insomnia, for example. If after two weeks nothing changes, they can try with the statin. Then with the diuretic. And so on.

It should be noted that there is no clinical trial to support this strategy. Clinical trials are usually made by adding drugs to treatments, not taking them away, because they are expensive studies that are often funded by companies or products. And what motivation can a company have to prove that it is better to prescribe fewer drugs instead of more?

But, although there are no studies to support it, withdrawing a beta blocker for two weeks, and then a diuretic another two, is an acceptable risk for a stable patient to take.

Experience shows that many of these patients—not all, unfortunately—can regain their sexual function. Then when they return for a medical appointment, what they express most is appreciation. "Doctor," they say, "you saved me." And they do not say it because of the heart attack, but because of the erection.

THERE IS NO REASON TO GIVE UP JUST BECAUSE THE REST OF THE WORLD IGNORES IT OR DISAPPROVES OF IT AND HAS YET TO REALIZE THAT SEX AMONG OLDER PEOPLE IS PERFECTLY NORMAL.

So, do not be fooled by the prejudices of age. There are people that are perfectly happy without sexual activity, which is perfectly fine. But there are many others for whom sex remains important at all ages. There is no reason to give up just because the rest of the world ignores it or disapproves of it and has yet to realize that sex among older people is perfectly normal.

Interest in Sex Remains High Even at Advanced Ages

Percentage of men who have orgasms

50 to 59 years old
Number of orgasms a month

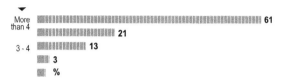

More
than 4   61
                  21
3 - 4   13
                  3
                  %

60 to 69 years old
Number of orgasms a month

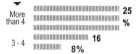

More
than 4   25
                  %
3 - 4   16
                  8%

70 to 79 years old
Number of orgasms a month

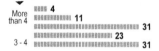

More
than 4   4
                  11
                  31
3 - 4   23
                  31

Percentage of men for whom the ability to
have orgasms is important or very important

From 50
to 59
years
 91%

60
to 69
years
 63%

70
to 79
years
 47%

Percentage of men who experience
sexual desire

From 50
to 59
years
 75%

In 60
to 69
years
 48%

In 70
to 79
years
 31%

Results of a study conducted in
Stockholm (Sweden) with a sample of
458 men representing the general
population, Source: *Age and Ageing*

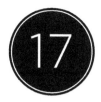

EAT WELL, LIVE LONGER

THE RELATIONSHIP BETWEEN DIET AND LONGEVITY

Making recommendations regarding a diet is easy. It is also complicated.

It is easy because many studies have been conducted to analyze what types of diet and food groups to choose from and what nutrients are related to better or worse health. We have enough data to know what works in general.

However, it is complicated because each person is a world unto themselves. What is suitable for one may not be for another. If your neighbor tells you "I have done well eliminating gluten from my diet" or "I take vitamin D supplements," this does not mean that you should go and do the same. It will depend on how one's body reacts to gluten or if there is a vitamin D deficiency. General recommendations can be made that are valid for the entire healthy population. But if you want detailed recommendations to solve individual problems, you must get a personalized recommendation.

An added difficulty is that, even when we know what works, many times we do not exactly know why it works. It is not that we do not have any idea and just go in blindly; we are not that ignorant. We have a few convincing general ideas and some good hypotheses to work from. However, when we do try and go into detail on what happens in our cells and how it affects our health, the human body is so complex and the variables that intermingle in nutrition are so numerous that it is impossible to be clear. For example, whether a food is better because it is an antioxidant or because it is anti-inflammatory: the most honest thing is to say that today we do not know exactly.

In the following pages, therefore, do not expect absolute answers or a universal solution for all cases. That solution, unfortunately, does not exist. But we will explain what works on a general level, why it helps to keep us healthy, and how it delays the aging process.

A first general principle, often overlooked, is that when we talk about nutrition it is useful to differentiate between quantity and quality. Ideally, of course, one should eat appropriate food in adequate quantities. But when we deviate from the ideal, we tend to confuse quantity problems with quality problems. This is something that is often observed in a consultation with a cardiologist. The patient asks, "Doctor, is eating potatoes bad?"

Well, the problem is not that you eat potatoes. The problem is that you eat too many potatoes. The problem is excess. There is no need to eliminate potatoes from your diet. Just eat less.

Let us begin with quantity. There is no need to insist that excess weight is harmful to your health. It is well known that obesity increases the risk of premature death due to myocardial infarction and stroke. It is less well known, but equally true, that the risk of at least eight different types of cancer is increased, including some of the more common ones, such as breast and colorectal cancer. It is known that obesity dangerously elevates levels of cholesterol, blood pressure, metabolic syndrome, diabetes, and osteoarthritis, one of the diseases that most limits the quality of life in the elderly.

But even if an obese person is free from all these ills, they will not be able to avoid aging faster than if they were the proper weight. Note that among the people who reach very advanced ages, say ninety-five and older, those of thin constitution predominate. Almost none are obese.

This has a biological explanation. The type of fat that accumulates in obesity, called white fat, secretes harmful molecules. These molecules are released into the blood and cause a state of inflammation in the body. It is a mild but chronic inflammation. It is hard to tell because no immediate damage is detected. One does not wake up one day and think, "My JNK protein is acting up today" or "I have an interleukin problem" or "The adipose tissue macrophages are really failing me."

Everything is stealthier. The white fat is very sneaky and does not call attention to itself, aside from its volume. It is not in a hurry, but neither does it rest. Nothing seems to change overnight, but year after year, the damage accumulates. We have already seen in chapter 15 that inflammation accelerates aging and that there is even the term *inflammaging*. This is exactly what white fat causes: aging by inflammation.

The first piece of advice we can give you on how to stop the aging process is to diet and avoid excess weight. There will be more in the following pages, but if there is only one piece of advice you take from this chapter, take this one. It is the most important.

> The first piece of advice we can give you on how to stop the aging process is to diet and avoid excess weight.

If obesity accelerates the aging process, is it possible that thinness can slow it down? After all, Alvise Cornaro, the Venetian nobleman we introduced you to in chapter 13, reached 102 living on 350 grams of food and two glasses of wine a day. We do not know how much he weighed, but it could not have been much.

Cornaro attributed his wellbeing and longevity to austerity. Apparently it worked for him, but we do not recommend that you do the same thing. If you take him as a role model, it is more likely that you will suffer malnutrition. You will deprive yourself of some important nutrient and your health will get worse instead of improving.

This is what we know today from the studies that explore how dietary restrictions can help prolong longevity. These studies offer spectacular results in laboratory animals. When the diet of C. elegans worms was restricted—a favorite of biologists because they are easy to experiment on—their longevity was prolonged by more than 50 percent. When they limited calories in fruit flies, another biologist's favorite, similar results were obtained.

If these examples do not convince you because you do not identify with invertebrates, we can also offer you data regarding mammals. When rats and mice are starved, it lengthens their life by up to 40 percent. At 40 percent, if extrapolated to people, that means people currently in their eighties will reach 110. Not bad, right?

The problem is that one cannot extrapolate to people so easily. All these studies indicate that caloric restriction extends life because it modifies the metabolism. In particular, it modulates the activity of molecules such as FOXO3, mTOR, or AMPK, which at this point may sound familiar after having been discussed in several chapters. Thus, caloric restriction reduces inflammation and improves activity of stem cells, as well as the ability to eliminate autophagy regenerative waste (the cleaning process of the cells explained in chapter 4). In fact, we are also interested in reducing inflammation and improving the autophagy and the activity of the stem cells. We want to modulate all these molecules that regulate the metabolism and that control the aging process. But each species has a different metabolism. A polar bear, who can go without eating while hibernation during the winter months, is not the same as a human being. A small herbivore such as a koala is not the same as a large carnivore such as a jaguar. We are all mammals, and yet we are all different.

If we review the data available on the human species, the relationship between weight and health draws a curve in the form of an arc. The center of the arc—the highest point where health and life expectancy reach their maximum—corresponds to a moderate weight. For a person who is 5'8", man or woman, the highest point of the arc is between 128 and 148 pounds. For a person who is six feet tall, it would be between 143 and 165 pounds.

If we move away from the center of the arc due to excess weight, we already know that our health will suffer and that life expectancy will diminish. But if we move away from it because of being underweight, it also has negative effects.

The human body needs a minimum of proteins, vitamins, calcium, iron, sodium...pretty much all nutrients that are vital to function. We are not like the polar bear who can endure several months without eating. We are more like a motorbike with a small tank that needs to be refueled as soon as it spends its fuel.

If you begin to deprive yourself of essential nutrients, you will find yourself with anemia due to iron deficiency; osteoporosis and higher risk of fractures due to lack of calcium; immune deficiency that will expose you to a greater risk of infections; more difficulty recovering from illness or injury; risk of cardiac arrhythmias; and, if you want to have children, risk of infertility. And, with all due respect to Alvise Cornaro, a high risk of premature death.

BEGIN TO MAKE CUTS IN ESSENTIAL NUTRIENTS AND YOU
MIGHT FIND YOURSELF WITH ANEMIA, OSTEOPOROSIS
AND A HIGHER RISK OF FRACTURES DUE TO LACK
OF CALCIUM, AND IMMUNE DEFICIENCY THAT WILL
EXPOSE YOU TO A GREATER RISK OF INFECTIONS.

So far, we have talked about the role of quantity in the diet. Now that we are going to talk about nutrients, and not only calories and weight, we will go into the issue of quality. Here is the million-dollar question, for those of us interested in the science of long life: is there any type of diet or any nutrient that can stop the aging process, or at least some aspects of the aging process?

Do not expect miracles, but these diets and nutrients exist.

Pay close attention to fats, which for most people are the most important variable. Some, such as the omega 3 fats that abound in fish, are beneficial. This was discovered in the Inuit population, who had little cardiovascular disease despite a diet composed almost exclusively of fish. This diet was later confirmed in the rest of the world. Omega 3 fats are healthy for the heart and arteries and are an essential component of the neuronal membrane. This suggests that omega 3 probably protects against cognitive decline, in part because it promotes a healthy blood flow to the brain and in part because of its direct action on neurons. It should be noted that until now no study has conclusively demonstrated this protective effect of omega 3.

Monounsaturated fats, which abound in olive oil, dried fruit, and certain nuts, including walnuts, almonds, and hazelnuts, have been associated with lower risk of chronic disease and greater longevity.

On the other hand, saturated fats in red meat have the opposite effect. If consumed in moderation, they pose no problem, but in excess, they are detrimental to cardiovascular health and accelerate the deterioration of the body.

Beyond fats, polyphenols deserve a special mention. They abound in fruits and vegetables, as well as in other plant-derived products, such as coffee and dark chocolate. Polyphenols are a large group of molecules, very varied, produced by the plants to protect them from aggressions such as the sun's ultraviolet radiation. They have an antioxidant effect and have been attributed benefits such as the prevention of cancers, diabetes, osteoporosis, and neurodegenerative and cardiovascular diseases.

It is not difficult to have a diet rich in polyphenols. Include an abundance of fruit and vegetables and remember that there are multiple different polyphenols of different colors and properties, so colorful salads are preferable to monochromatic salads.

But bear in mind that some polyphenols inhibit the absorption of iron by the body. Therefore, if a person has iron deficiency anemia, which is the most common, it is preferable that the person avoid the polyphenols in meals that include food rich in iron, such as red meat or tuna, as well as when taking iron supplements.

An anti-aging diet should also be rich in fiber, which is found in fruit, legumes, vegetables, and whole grains. This is because fiber is beneficial for the intestinal microbiota, which is the whole of microorganisms that live in our intestines. Microbiota is essential to the functioning of the immune system. And we already know that a good immune system not only helps fight infections and eliminate cancerous and precancerous cells, but also modulates inflammation that could lead to accelerated aging.

Our diet must be scarce in salt and sugar. Scarce does not mean prohibited. Salt and sugar are necessary, even indispensable to the human body. If we like both those things so much, it is because they are vital, and evolution has endowed us with a sense of taste that particularly appreciates sweet and savory flavors. From sugar, we get energy to feed our organs, particularly the brain, which is a voracious consumer of glucose. From salt we get sodium, on which approximately 30 trillion cells in the body depend.

But evolution made us appreciate salt and sugar in contexts where these were scarce. In the African savannah, where human beings evolved for most of history, it was not easy to get sugar or salt. Now we are in the opposite situation, in an era of nutritional abundance unprecedented in the history of mankind.

Just a few numbers might give you an idea of the anomaly that we are living. The human genus—or *Homo* genus— appeared in Africa about 2.8 million years ago. The anatomy and behavior evolved towards a bigger brain and more advanced technologies until our species appeared, *Homo sapiens*, not more than 200,000 years ago, which represents the most recent 10 percent of human history.

We lived the nomadic life; we organized ourselves into small groups of hunter-gatherers that woke up every day without knowing what food would be found, until agriculture was invented some 10,000 years ago, in the final 5 percent of the history of our species.

And from agriculture we developed cooking, commerce, production surplus, and in the last century, industrial food, supermarkets, restaurant chains—the economy of abundance. Therefore, of the 10,000 years of agriculture history, only in the last one hundred—the last 1 percent—has there been this excess of salts, sugars, and saturated fats.

If we put all these figures in perspective, the result is that only in the last 0.005 percent of the history of mankind have we found ourselves facing a situation of an oversupply of food. It is such a small percentage that it is difficult to understand how small of a percentage it is. It is one part in 20,000. Barely a blink in our long human history.

This presents quite a challenge for us. Life in the bush taught us to survive in scarcity and succumb to the temptations of abundance. But modern economies offer us a myriad of temptations in the form of food, distractions, and even addictions. Of course, it is preferable to have food than to be malnourished or starving. We are not against progress. But we must learn to live with abundance in a way that does not harm us; this is a problem for which evolution has not prepared us.

Fortunately, there is a type of diet that solves this problem. It is a diet rich in the nutrients that we said helps stop the aging process. These are the monounsaturated fats, omega 3 fats, fiber, and polyphenols. Such a diet does not abuse salts, sugars, or saturated fats. It is a varied diet that provides all the necessary vitamins and minerals, which help to prevent some problems associated with the aging process, such as the risk of fractures due to lack of calcium. It is generous in plant-based foods, such as fruits and vegetables, and scarce in red meat and processed foods. And it has the great advantage of being organized in a structured schedule with breakfast, lunch, and dinner, plus one or two snacks throughout the day, usually eaten as a family or in company. Hunger pangs that may lead to binge eating can be avoided, and this diet has the additional benefits of social interaction.

This is the diet followed by the centenarians of the islands of Ikaria and Sardinia mentioned in chapter 8. It is the diet that Jeanne Calment followed. It is, as you may have already guessed, the Mediterranean diet.

If you are skeptical, you might be interested to know that the Mediterranean diet is one of the few whose impact on health has been evaluated in clinical trials. The benefits of the Mediterranean diet are no longer just an attractive hypothesis derived from common sense; it is a diet that contains healthy ingredients, and Mediterranean populations have been shown to have a high life expectancy.

There are proven benefits that have been evaluated in the same way we evaluate pharmaceutical drugs: in large clinical trials in which some volunteers had a healthy diet—as healthy as possible, but not Mediterranean—and others had a Mediterranean diet, rich in olive oil and dry fruit.

The results are unequivocal. After five years in a clinical trial involving 7,447 volunteers over fifty-five years of age, the rate of heart attacks, strokes, and cardiovascular deaths was 30 percent lower among those who followed the Mediterranean diet than those who had a healthy diet. The cognitive decline associated with age was also lower among the Mediterranean diet group. Among women, the rate of breast cancer was also lower with the Mediterranean diet.

Another study, based on retrospective data of 90,000 women in the United States, noted that those who followed a diet similar to the Mediterranean diet had a lower risk of bone fractures due to osteoporosis.

> For now, with what we know today, you will not find a better diet than the Mediterranean diet to live a longer, healthier life.

It should be noted that we do not know everything about the relationship between diet and aging. This is a dynamic field of research and, within a few years, maybe not too many, recommendations will be made based on new studies. It is possible that the studies on caloric restriction will reveal in the future how to improve health and prolong life with a more frugal diet. It is possible that a period of fasting is beneficial. Or the discovery of some unexpected benefits that we do not see today of some nutrient or food groups, just as we discovered in the recent past the benefits of fats deriving from olive oil, dried fruit, and fish. All these research topics are open. But for now, with what we know in the year 2018, you will not find a better diet than the Mediterranean diet to live a longer, healthier life.

The Staple Foods of the Mediterranean Diet

FOOD OF PLANT ORIGIN

Predominant in the Mediterranean diet

Olive oil

Provides
monounsaturated fats

Fruit, legumes, and vegetables

Consumed daily in
abundance. Provide
valuable micronutrients

Dried fruit

Provides
polyunsaturated fats
and micronutrients

Cereals, rice, potatoes, vegetables

Complex carbohydrates
are the basis of the first meal
and the main source of energy

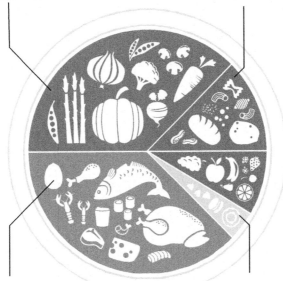

OTHER

The Mediterranean diet
is a flexible diet in
which no food is
forbidden. But some,
such as sweets must
be consumed with
moderation

FOOD OF ANIMAL ORIGIN

Chicken and pork

The most common meats in
the Mediterranean diet

Veal

Rich in iron, but due to its
high content of saturated fats,
consumption should only be
occasional

Dairy products and eggs

Provide protein and
micronutrients

Fish and seafood

Provide polyunsaturated fats
and should be consumed
several times a week.

BEVERAGES

Water
should be the main
drink in any diet

Red wine
in moderation is
healthy. In excess
is harmful

ANTIOXIDANTS AND FREE RADICALS

HOW TO AVOID THE ACCUMULATION OF TOXIC SUBSTANCES IN THE CELLS

At the end of the previous chapter, we told you that we do not know the whole story about the relationship between antioxidants and aging. One of the things that we do not yet understand is where exactly antioxidants fit in.

If we were to ask you if antioxidants are beneficial or harmful to your health, particularly against aging, you would probably say they are beneficial. If we were to ask you about free radicals, you would probably say they are harmful. However, we are not so sure.

We will summarize what we know today about the relationship between antioxidants and aging and you will see that things are not so black and white. There is no army of noble Jedi knights in antioxidant uniforms fighting against the clone army of free radicals. We have an intricate plot with complex characters that are either good or evil, depending on the details of each scene. This is a plot worthier of Shakespeare than George Lucas.

The action began in 1956, when Denham Harman presented the first version of his theory on aging based on free radicals. Although some of Harman's ideas turned out flawed, he was an extraordinary scientist. He was the first to interpret the aging process as a biochemical problem and to search for strategies to counter it.

He trained as a chemist and began his career in the oil industry. It was there that he started to study the reactions of free radicals. Things went well. While working for Shell Oil, he developed thirty-five patents, including a compound used for years on plastic adhesive strips to catch flies.

Harman could have been rich had he stayed with Shell. But he had a restless mind. As he began to reflect on the aging process, he had this great idea that its causes could be investigated to develop effective treatments. Today this idea seems obvious, but in Harman's era it was visionary.

There was no guarantee of success. Still, he left his promising career as a chemist and enrolled at Stanford University in California to study medicine. He finished his studies in 1954, when he was thirty-eight years old. He later became director of cardiovascular research at the University of Nebraska Medical Center.

His theory of free radicals was initially met with skepticism, if not outright indifference. His idea was that free radicals are molecules that cause chemical reactions within the cells and that these reactions can be harmful. So harmful, according to Harman, that he considered this the main cause of aging.

If you are interested in the chemical details, here is a summary. Free radicals are molecules deprived of an electron. Free radicals are very unstable and react quickly with other compounds, trying to capture the needed electron to gain stability. Generally, free radicals attack the nearest stable molecule, stealing its electron. When the attacked molecule loses its electron, it becomes a free radical itself, triggering a domino effect within the cells that can lead to grave consequences.

The problem, Harman noted, is that any cell in the human body generates free radicals. It generates them because it consumes oxygen to produce energy, which creates a type of free radical called reactive oxygen species (ROS).

Free radicals are, therefore, a by-product of breathing—a side effect to being alive.

Free radicals are also generated in response to aggressions such as the sun's UV radiation, toxins in tobacco, and air pollutants.

Not all radicals are small criminals happy to recover their lost electron and then rehabilitate. Some—such as the superoxide radical, with a name worthy of a comic book villain, or the hydroxyl radical, which is equally evil—create organized crime networks and sow chaos inside the cells. They can damage DNA, oxidize amino acids, oxidize fats, shorten telomeres, and interfere with chemical reactions necessary for an effective government of the cell.

Luckily, we have antidotes. If the ROS are molecules that trigger harmful oxidation reactions, there are other types of molecules that can counteract them. They are the antioxidants—the heroes of the comic book. Hence the idea that a diet rich in antioxidants can be beneficial for our health or that cosmetics that incorporate antioxidants can delay the aging of the skin.

This theory is plausible. There is some empirical data supporting it. The first observation is that, as we get older, we have more free radicals in our cells. But this does not prove that free radicals cause aging. It could be the opposite—that the aging process causes the accumulation of free radicals. Or that they are a cause-and-reaction phenomena, one causing the other. Or that they occur in parallel without any relationship between them. As you can see, when two phenomena coincide, such as aging and the accumulation of free radicals, it is not easy to clarify if there is a cause-effect relationship.

The second observation, which we have already mentioned, is that free radicals damage DNA and other important components of the cells. This is what led Harman to think that free radicals are the cause and aging the result.

He experimented with mice to test this theory, exposing them to ionizing radiation to generate large amounts of free radicals and then giving them high doses of antioxidants to see the effect. He proved that antioxidants lengthened the average life of mice. According to the type of antioxidant used, life expectancy was increased between 30 and 45 percent, compared to the mice that received radiation but no antioxidants. These are spectacular percentages.

These experiments might look fairly convincing. If antioxidants prolong life, then free radicals shorten it and must be the cause of aging, right?

Not necessarily. Note that Harman experimented with

mice exposed to ionizing radiation. Also note that it extended their average life, not the maximum longevity. His experiments were the equivalent to infecting animals with the plague, then giving them antibiotics. The animals that received the treatment lived longer, but of course, this does not mean that antibiotics delay the aging process. And it does not mean that data from a sample of severely ill animals can be applied to healthy people.

It is a reminder that we must be careful when drawing conclusions from experiments. Even more so when there are commercial interests involved, as in the case of antioxidants.

In fact, when considering the collection of empirical data, the theory of free radicals as the cause of aging must be refined. Mice genetically engineered to have more free radicals in their cells, contrary to what might be expected, do not age faster. In yeast and worms, free radicals may even prolong life rather than shorten it.

If you prefer an example from the human body, think about what happens when you pursue physical activity. The more activity, the more consumption of oxygen and therefore the more production of free radicals in the cells. Exercise, thus, should be a highly toxic activity that shortens life. However, it is a healthy activity that lengthens it. How do you explain that?

If Harman had been an evolutionary scientist as well as a chemist and doctor, he would have been inspired by Darwin more than Mendeleev, and he might have asked himself how the cells adapted to their own free radicals. Because there is no doubt that free radicals can be harmful. We have already seen that they can degrade the DNA and proteins. But in nature, there is no good and evil. What is poison for the tiger is defense for the cobra. Like the yin and yang, all that harms can also protect and all that protects can also harm. If Harman had reasoned like Darwin, perhaps he would have asked himself how our cells protect themselves from their own toxins just as the snake protects itself from its own venom. And knowing that everything in nature is recycled and reused, he would have also asked himself if the cells had invented some way to benefit from these free radicals.

The answers are provided by experiments carried out in recent years, which indicate that free radicals participate effectively in chemical reactions necessary for the proper functioning of the cells.

Because an excess of free radicals is damaging, the cells generate their own antioxidants to neutralize them. Thus, when facing small daily aggressions, such as those derived from respiration during physical activity, the cell activates protective mechanisms. In fact, these small assaults may even be beneficial, according to a currently popular idea known as mitohormesis.

In line with this theory, it is the free radicals themselves that have an anti-aging effect, since they are the starting point of many desirable biochemical reactions in the cell. In a nutshell, this is how it goes: the free radicals activate the p38 MAPK protein, which regulates the Nrf2 protein in the nucleus of the cell, which has an antioxidant effect, which then promotes an increase in longevity.

But they are double-edged swords. Massive attacks of free radicals are harmful and overwhelm the defense ability of the cells. It is what happened to the irradiated mice in Harman's experiments. And it is what happens in tissues of the human body when we punish them ruthlessly, like skin when it suffers sunburn or lungs when we fill them with pollutants.

At this point, one might think that if antioxidants are protectors, a diet rich in antioxidants would be beneficial. The problem is that no one has proven that a diet rich in antioxidants increases longevity. This may surprise you. It has at least surprised those investigators who have examined the potential benefits of antioxidants and found the results to be underwhelming. How do you explain it?

We do not know for sure. As we explained at the beginning of the chapter, we do not have all the answers on antioxidants. But we have a good hypothesis: if a cell already produces the antioxidants it needs, it does not do any good to give it more. It is like giving food to someone who is not hungry. It could even be that filling the cells with antioxidants may inhibit the natural defense mechanisms of protection. We are in the uncertain terrain of the hypothesis.

If you are a fan of antioxidants and all of this does not sound very convincing, there is an important study conducted in Finland among male smokers that may dampen your enthusiasm. The study was based on a sample of 29,133 smokers over the age of fifty, with a high risk of developing lung cancer. They were offered vitamin E and beta-carotene supplements in the hope of reducing the risk. Some only took vitamin E, others took only beta-carotene, some took both, and others took neither. The result was the opposite of what the researchers expected: beta-carotene supplements increased the risk of lung cancer by 18 percent, and vitamin E decreased it.

Of course, this does not mean that antioxidants must be eradicated. It just means that the relationship between antioxidants and cancer is not simple and linear. It is wrong to say that the more antioxidants, the less cancer. It is a complex relationship; what is beneficial one moment may be harmful the next. Ultimately, it will depend on the type of antioxidant and the type of cancer cell.

In fact, excess free radicals have the opposite effect in

the initiation and progression of cancer. Consequently, antioxidants can also have opposite effects.

In a precancerous cell, a high level of free radicals promotes accumulation of DNA damage and cancer cell conversion. It is what happened to Harman's irradiated mice: the extra antioxidants had a protective effect.

But once cancer has begun, tumor cells are characterized by having many free radicals that lead to self-destruction and need many antioxidants to survive. In this case, the extra dose of some—not all—antioxidants may be helpful for tumor cells but harmful to the person.

If instead of clarifying things, we have confused you, welcome to the gray zone of uncertainty. The situation is truly confusing. Unfortunately, nothing is simple in the human body, and if someone promises you easy solutions, be wary. Uncertainty is the scientist's area of expertise, which means there is a whole field of questions that have not yet found answers.

There will come a day in the future, possibly not very distant, where the fog surrounding antioxidants will be lifted and clear recommendations will be made, just like we can today in treating infections.

> What we can recommend is a varied diet, rich in antioxidants—like the Mediterranean diet, since it is beneficial for the maintenance of good health, reducing the risk of some cancers and delaying the aging process.

With infections, there was also a period of confusion when we could not distinguish virus from bacteria, or even know what bacteria was. The same will happen with free radicals and antioxidants. We will clear the unknowns; it is only a matter of time.

What we can recommend in the meantime is a varied diet that is rich in antioxidants—like the Mediterranean diet, since it is beneficial for maintaining good health, reducing the risk of some cancers and delaying the aging process. In the previous chapter, we told you that polyphenols in fruit, legumes, and vegetables—which form part of the plant's defense system—consumed through diet, are considered beneficial. There are also beneficial polyphenols from cocoa, coffee, and red wine, if taken in moderation. The beta-carotene in carrots and other carotenoids are also antioxidants and do not increase, but rather reduce, the risk of lung cancer when consumed as part of a diet.

FROM THE MOMENT WE SUBSTITUTE THE ANTIOXIDANTS
ON OUR PLATE WITH ANTIOXIDANTS FROM A MEDICINE
CABINET—TAKEN AS PILLS AND NOT VEGETABLES,
CHANGING THE DOSE AND THE INTERACTIONS BETWEEN
THEM SINCE WE ARE TAKING PURIFIED ANTIOXIDANTS
AND NOT IN COMBINATION WITH OTHER NUTRIENTS—
THESE RECOMMENDATIONS ARE NO LONGER VALID.

But from the moment we substitute the antioxidants in the food with antioxidants from a medicine cabinet—taken as pills instead of eating vegetables, changing the dose and the interactions between them since we are taking purified antioxidants and not in combination with other nutrients—these recommendations stop being valid. We would love to tell you that there are antioxidants pills that help preserve health and delay the aging process. Unfortunately, there are none for now.

Free Radicals and Antioxidants, a Complex Relationship

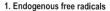 Free radicals O Antioxidants

1. Endogenous free radicals
The mitochondria produce energy in the cells and release free radicals

6. Excess
Too many antioxidants in the diet can prevent the cell from fulfilling its role, which would be detrimental

2. Exogenous free radicals
External stimuli that create free radicals (radiation, toxins...)

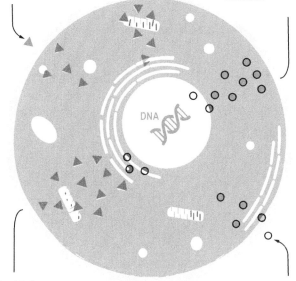

3. Harmful effects
An excess of free radicals is damaging to the cells and affects the DNA

4. Endogenous antioxidants
In the presence of free radicals, the nucleus of the cells activates the production of antioxidants

5. Exogenous antioxidants
The antioxidants in the diet help counteract free radicals

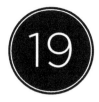

YOUTH PILLS

WHY THERE ARE NO ANTI-AGING DRUGS NOW, BUT THERE WILL BE IN THE FUTURE

If there were a pill that extended life, would you take it? Would you take a drug with acceptable side effects and an affordable price that increases life expectancy by one or two decades, maybe more?

A pill like that may sound like science fiction. This is something more appropriate for the happy world of Aldous Huxley or the future imagined by Arthur C. Clarke than for a science article. But, as crazy as that idea may seem, there are researchers and pharmaceutical companies that have begun to work on making this a reality. They are investing time and money because they believe that it is possible to create this kind of pill.

At the time of this writing, there are at least fourteen US pharmaceutical companies working to create drugs that combat the aging process. This pill's main purpose is not to prolong life but to enhance the years lived in good health and reduce the years lived with suffering. There are two other drugs that have been used for years for other purposes but appear to have the side effect of prolonging health and longevity.

Of course, not all the innovative drugs that are in development will reach fruition. It is possible that some will not be as effective as expected, or will have unacceptable side effects, or will not receive the necessary investment to move forward. In pharmacological research, just as in the Gospel according to St. Matthew, many are called and few are chosen.

But these different molecules being investigated as potential anti-aging drugs have something in common. All of them are based on solid scientific data. We still do not know about the biology of longevity, as we have explained in previous chapters. But the new therapies being developed are not the product of opportunistic charlatans that promise eternal youth. They are the result of what has been discovered in recent decades about how the human body changes with age. This is not a guarantee of success, but it is a good starting point.

The idea that it is possible to modulate longevity with a drug in mammals like us was demonstrated in 2009 when a US research team reported the results of their experiments on mice. The mice were treated with rapamycin when they were twenty months old—equivalent to a person at age sixty—and it was discovered that the drug extended their life by 14 percent in females and 9 percent in males.

It had been observed that rapamycin prolongs life in yeast, flies, and worms as early as 2003, but never had it been shown that it could have the same effect in our class of vertebrates.

Shortly after, it was observed that, if the treatment starts when the mice are nine months old instead of waiting until their twenties, the effect is even more dramatic: life lasts, on average, about 25 percent longer. If this result were repeated in people, this would mean that the average life expectancy in Spain could increase from the current eighty-three years to about 105.

THE NEW THERAPIES ARE NOT PRODUCTS OF
OPPORTUNISTIC CHARLATANS THAT PROMISE
ETERNAL YOUTH. THEY ARE THE RESULT OF WHAT
HAS BEEN DISCOVERED IN RECENT DECADES
ABOUT HOW THE HUMAN BODY CHANGES WITH
AGE. THIS IS NOT A GUARANTEE OF SUCCESS,
BUT IT IS A GOOD STARTING POINT.

And these additional years will be lived in good health:
the mice treated with rapamycin had less cancer, less
obesity, and fewer symptoms of Alzheimer's than those
that did not receive the drug.

With this data, one might think that rapamycin should
be tried on people. But this type of research requires
patience if you want to do it well and avoid disappoint-
ments. Rapamycin is a special drug that was discovered
in bacteria on Easter Island. Hence its name, because
Easter Island is called Rapa Nui in the local language. It
has been used for decades in people who have received
transplants because it has an immunosuppressive effect.
It is also used in people who are implanted with a stent
in the heart, because it inhibits the proliferation of the
cells and prevents the arteries from closing again. It is
also used for the treatment of certain kidney, pancreatic,
and breast cancers. But it is not free from side effects.

Precisely because rapamycin inhibits the defense mechanisms of the immune system as well as the proliferation of the cells, among other effects, it is ethically questionable that it can be offered to healthy people to prolong and improve life, since it could also have the opposite effect: make it worse and shorten it. We can accept that a drug has important side effects when treating people with a serious illness, but not when treating people who are perfectly healthy.

An additional problem is that we do not yet have any reliable and agreed-upon techniques to measure the rate at which we age, so we should wait decades to see if rapamycin truly does extend life in people.

How do we solve these issues and move forward in the investigation of rapamycin to obtain safe and effective anti-aging drugs? First, by looking for a technique that accurately indicates the rate of aging: the biomarker. Perhaps the telomeres will be used in the future as biomarkers of aging. There are already groups working on this line of research. But for now, we have no way of measuring whether a drug has any effect on the rate of aging.

Secondly, the rapamycin should be tested on animals that are more like people than mice. The experiments with mice are useful because they have a similar biology to ours, they are easy to breed and cheap to feed in a lab, and they have short lives; therefore, results are fast. But there is always the doubt that the results seen in mice will be replicated in humans.

To dispel this doubt as much as possible, there is an ongoing study led by the University of Washington to test rapamycin on dogs, which offer the advantage of living in the same environments as people. And the first results of a treatment with rapamycin in marmoset monkeys—which are primates like us—have been released, and the results so far are positive.

And finally, scientists are looking for a molecule inspired by rapamycin with fewer side effects. It is known that rapamycin inhibits the mTOR protein, which you may remember from chapter 13. We told you then that mTOR regulates body growth and reduces longevity. Therefore, it is not surprising that lifespan is increased when mTOR is blocked.

One important detail we have not mentioned before is that mTOR activates two groups of different proteins. They are called, in the jargon of molecular biology, mTORC1 and mTORC2, and have different effects in the body. Rapamycin, logically, affects both groups of proteins. But while its beneficial effects on the aging process are based mainly on mTORC1, its unwanted side effects are based mostly on mTORC2. For this reason, if we obtain a drug to continue to act on mTORC1 but leave the mTORC2 proteins alone, it could retain most of its efficacy against aging while avoiding most side effects.

We have good reason to believe that such a drug would be efficient. Rapamycin regulates autophagy, the cell's cleaning mechanism we explained in chapter 4. It promotes the maintenance of progenitor cells and regenerates tissues. It stimulates the AMPK molecule, which is the one that activates when we exercise, if you remember chapter 13. It moderates inflammation reactions that accelerate aging. All of them behave in a manner similar to caloric restriction; in other words, they force the body to devote resources to maintenance and give up on growth. That is the great advantage of austerity. One stops being distracted by luxuries and focuses on the essentials.

As you can see, the research to obtain an antidote against the aging process is in progress. Not only is it in progress, but it is gaining momentum, fast.

There are other options besides rapamycin. There is another drug that has also been used for years and seems able to extend the number of years lived in good health. If you have diabetic family members, you may have heard of it. It is metformin, which has become the most prescribed drug in the world for people with type 2 diabetes.

Like rapamycin, metformin prolongs life in worms and certain types of mice, though the same result has not been observed in flies or rats. It also acts in a way that simulates caloric restriction, although with some differences that explain why its effects are not the same.

But metformin offers a major advantage over rapamycin. It has been used for sixty years and is taken by many more people; therefore, there is much more accumulated data. It is considered a very safe drug; researchers have been able to retrospectively analyze its effects on longevity. Researchers at the University of Cardiff in the United Kingdom revised the data of 78,000 diabetics treated with metformin, then compared them to 12,000 diabetics treated with another drug called sulfonylurea, and to 90,000 healthy people.

As expected, it was confirmed that longevity is greater among diabetic patients taking metformin than among those who did not. Specifically, the statistical analysis suggests that survival is 62 percent greater in the first group. What is most extraordinary is that, despite being diabetic, their survival rate is higher than that of the general population: 18 percent higher.

Still, a retrospective study with data on diabetics is not sufficient proof that metformin extends life and delays the aging process for the general population. To find this out, it is necessary to conduct a study for people who are not diabetic and must be prospective.

This study is already in progress. The TAME study (Targeting Aging with Metformin), is being conducted with 3,000 people between the ages of seventy and eighty in the United States. In the absence of a biomarker to measure the aging process, studies will investigate whether metformin protects against cardiovascular diseases, cancers, and cognitive decline. The results are expected early in the next decade.

For now, the prospects are good. No one dares to devote five years of his career to a clinical trial, as in the case of Nir Barzilai from the Albert Einstein College of Medicine in New York, if it isn't to discover something important.

Knowledge on the biology of aging has advanced enough in the last two decades for a whole range of molecules to emerge that are candidates for prolonging life and, above all, for prolonging the years lived in good health.

And no one would give him $50 million in funding, which is what TAME will cost, if they did not believe he can do it.

Beyond rapamycin and metformin, our knowledge about the biology of aging has advanced enough in the last two decades to have a whole range of candidate molecules to extend life and, above all, to extend the years lived in good health.

There is exploration of the enhancers for the FGF-21 protein, which—among other functions—activates the molecule AMPK, which we have already seen is beneficial. Or the CGRP molecule inhibitors, which increase with age and appear to promote aging, at least in mice. Or compounds that raise levels of coenzyme NAD+, which is essential for an efficient metabolism.

There are more examples; the list is extensive. It is impossible to know which of these experimental drugs will succeed and which will fail. Probably many will fail and few succeed. But these examples show that there are ongoing efforts to attack a problem that, until recently, was considered unapproachable. Instead of attacking diseases individually—which in the best of cases leads to avoiding one, just to fall into another—the goal now is to treat aging globally.

When this expectation is fulfilled, the consequences will be greater than if we eradicated all cancers or all strokes in one fell swoop. Because if no one died of cancer, the average life expectancy of the population would increase a little—three years and two months, according to calculations by Jay Olshansky of the University of Illinois in Chicago—since people would die shortly after from other causes. If no one died of myocardial infarction, the effect would be similar: three more years of life expectancy for women and three for men, according to Olshansky. But if we treat aging as a whole, we might be able to simultaneously prevent various diseases that increase with age, including cancer, cardiovascular, and neurodegenerative diseases. These increase life expectancy not just by a few years, but by decades.

But we have not yet reached this point, and the path will not be easy. Although there is growing enthusiasm for research on aging, remember the telling story of resveratrol. The name might sound familiar, since some of the anti-aging products sold today contain resveratrol.

This is a molecule that abounds in black grapes and red wine. In laboratory experiments conducted in 1997, it was discovered that it inhibits the formation and growth of tumors, which suggests that it could be useful for the prevention of some cancers. But since then, it has not been possible to demonstrate in people that following a diet rich in resveratrol or taking resveratrol supplements reduces the risk of any type of cancer.

In 2003, a team from Harvard University discovered that resveratrol activates sirtuins, which was viewed as a great advance in aging research. A big step forward and a great business opportunity. Sirtuins, as you may remember from chapter 3, are the cells' guardian angels. In mice, sirtuin 1 (SIRT1) extended their life by 44 percent. In Harvard University experiments, resveratrol had a similar effect on caloric restriction and extended life expectancy by 70 percent.

From these results, the pharmaceutical company Sirtris was founded with the objective of creating an anti-aging drug based on sirtuins. The perspective was so promising that the multinational company GlaxoSmithKline bought Sirtris in 2008 for $720 million. Eight years later, that investment has not yielded any results.

What can we learn from the story of resveratrol? At least a lesson in humility. It seemed that resveratrol activated sirtuins; it seemed that the sirtuins activated the caloric restriction program; and it seemed like this caloric restriction program extended life. It seemed so because it was what had been observed in experiments made with yeast under controlled conditions. They were well-executed experiments and the results are relevant. But for these results to translate into medical advances, the effects must also happen with people who do not live in the controlled conditions of yeast in a lab, but in more complex, diverse, and changing environments.

> The same way that cancer treatments we have today are the result of decades-long effort, we cannot expect treatments for aging to arrive tomorrow. But we can hope that they are not too far off in the future.

If we stop a moment to consider where we are, we will see that research on aging is at a point similar to where we were with cancer research thirty years ago. Even though our knowledge on aging is incomplete, the pieces are starting to come together and a vision of the whole is emerging for the first time. For now, it is just an outline.

It is clear that we are missing pieces of the puzzle, and since we do not know which pieces are missing, we cannot appreciate the extent of their importance. The problem is that we ignore the enormity of our ignorance.

But in the same way that cancer research has led to better treatments, to the point that today many cancers are now being overcome, it is foreseeable that research on aging will lead to more effective treatments to prolong the years lived in good health and to extend life. The same way that the treatments we have today for cancer are the result of decades-long effort—it has been forty years since the discovery of the first cancer genes in 1976—we cannot expect treatment for aging to get here tomorrow. But we can hope it is not too far off in the future.

The Human Body Adapts its Metabolism to Available Resources

●—Activates ├— Blocks ⬡ Main molecules involved ○ Drugs

WHEN RESOURCES ARE ABUNDANT
A sedentary lifestyle and an excessive diet create a situation of abundant resources

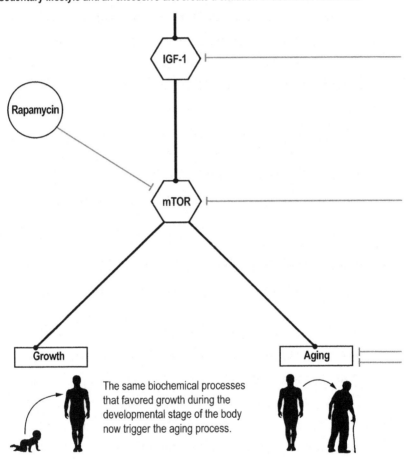

The same biochemical processes that favored growth during the developmental stage of the body now trigger the aging process.

WHEN RESOURCES ARE SCARCE
Physical activity and a moderate diet simulate a situation of scarce resources

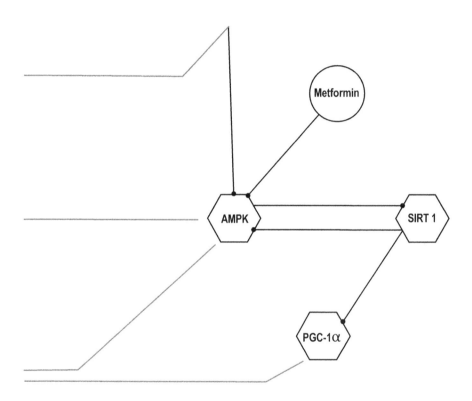

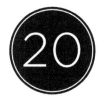

MOTIVATION: DIVINE TREASURE

BASIC PREVENTIVE MEASURES FOR A LONG AND HEALTHY LIFE

Not everything always goes as planned.

We can do everything right and the result can go wrong. In the time of Pierre-Simon Laplace, who said that by knowing the initial conditions of the universe the whole future could be predicted, and who thought that all effect has a cause, we could have blamed ourselves—or others—for the disappointing result.

But that was two hundred years ago. Today we see the universe through the eyes of the theoretical physicist Max Planck. We are in times of quantum indeterminacy. We know that there are elements of chance that can disrupt the best-laid plans and that, sometimes, no one is to blame.

Chance governs particles of the universe that obey seemingly absurd laws of quantum physics, forming the Sun and the Earth and life itself. It also affects living creatures, which cannot control everything that happens inside their body or all interactions with the external environment. The cancer that comes without reason, DNA mutations, the malaria-carrying mosquito, unexpected bacteria, a bolt of lightning that strikes, the connections formed in our neurons, the connections that are lost...All these are examples of what we call stochastic phenomena: unpredictable phenomena influenced by random variables.

This does not mean that we are defenseless against chance. Within the unpredictability, we have strategies to reduce the margin of uncertainty and increase control. Strategies to decide how we want to live. To close the door to undesired bacteria, to minimize damage in our DNA, to avoid accidents and ultimately enjoy a long and healthy life. We have written about strategies such as those in detail in previous chapters. Staying physically active, keeping the brain fit, preserving relationships, avoiding excess in our diet, managing stress, following our path and not those that others want...But even when we do all this, we are not safe from the unforeseen. We can be victims of stochastic damages. So, to all the recommendations we must add one more: do not neglect preventive measures and early diagnosis. And the number one recommendation, by far the most important one, is to not smoke. All of you, including those of you who smoke, know that tobacco is harmful. You know that it increases the risk of cancer; you know it is damaging to the cardiovascular system, that it increases the risk of heart attack and stroke; and you know that it increases respiratory diseases such as COPD, which has no cure and is the third leading cause of death in the world...There is no need to insist on it.

What you may not know is to what extent the risk increases. Because most smokers do not develop lung cancer, if you smoke, chances are you will not either, right? And most likely, if they smoke, they will not have a heart attack. So, why not light another cigarette? You can stop smoking another day. A few numbers might help put the issue in perspective.

Approximately one in six men who smoke will develop lung cancer, according to a study by the International Cancer Research Agency, based on data from six countries in Eastern Europe. An independent study conducted in Canada has reached the same result: one in six. It is possible that the figure is different in Spain or in other countries, because it can be influenced by variables such as the number of cigarettes a day, the age in which the smoker began to consume tobacco, or the way in which it is consumed. But we do not have comparable data from Spain, so we will keep one in six as the best approximation we have.

KEEPING PHYSICALLY ACTIVE, MAINTAINING A FIT BRAIN, TAKING CARE OF OUR RELATIONSHIPS, AVOIDING A DIET OF EXCESS, CONTROLLING STRESS, FOLLOWING OUR PATH AND NOT THE ONE OTHERS WANT US TO FOLLOW...BUT EVEN WHEN WE DO ALL THIS, WE ARE NOT SAFE FROM THE UNFORESEEN.

This means that, if you find a group of six people smoking outside a bar, one of them is likely to suffer from lung cancer. No one can know which of the six it will be. They may all get lucky and not get lung cancer. But it may also happen that they have bad luck and two get it. Or very bad luck and three may get it.

Now imagine for a moment a group of six people in front of a train track. They must cross it, and a train is approaching at full speed. Let us suppose that the probability that the train will hit them is one in six. If all six cross, one will die. If you were one of these six people, would you cross? Would you invite others to cross? If you were to see your partner, or your children, or any person that you care about ready to cross, would you try to stop them? This train represents tobacco. It hits with lung cancer one in six people that cross its path.

One of every six, if you want an idea of the magnitude of the risk, is the probability of dying from a bullet in a game of Russian roulette. There are six compartments for bullets in the cylinder of a revolver, a bullet is placed in one of them, the barrel is spun, and the gun is shot.

The other five smokers, who have crossed the track and have missed the train, are not yet safe. Keep in mind that carcinogenic compounds of tobacco smoke not only come into contact with the lungs, but also with other tissues vulnerable to cancer. For this reason, the vast majority of cancers of the larynx, esophagus, or oral cavity—among others—happen to smokers. Some of these compounds later go into the bloodstream and are distributed throughout the body, which can cause cancers of the bladder, kidney, and pancreas...In total, there are more than fifteen different types of cancer linked to smoking.

In the blood, as you know, tobacco compounds also affect the cardiovascular system, which cause a state of chronic inflammation in the blood vessels, increasing the risk of catastrophic damage in the form of heart attacks and stroke in the brain.

In the lungs, respiratory capacity is stealthily reduced even before the smoker realizes it, and over time, the capacity for physical activity is reduced.

It is not easy to calculate the total cancer, cardiovascular, and respiratory damage caused by tobacco. There are people who smoke for decades and apparently suffer no damage without anyone being able to explain why. Jeanne Calment smoked, if you remember, for ninety-six years, and this did not stop her from becoming the world's longest-living person. Other people, however, are highly vulnerable to tobacco, but do not discover it until it is too late.

To estimate the total bill, researches at the Harvard School of Public Health analyzed data of more than 100,000 women in the United States, collected over twenty-five years. There were 12,483 deaths recorded during this period, which allowed the comparison of mortality between smokers and those that abstained.

Once the data was processed, it was discovered that 64 percent of smokers had died prematurely from tobacco-related damage. Sixty-four percent is approximately two out of every three. That is much more dangerous than playing Russian roulette.

Another research group has calculated, also from US data, how much smoking shortens life. They found that, in women, the likelihood of reaching eighty years of age is 70 percent without smoking, but is reduced to 38 percent if they smoke. In men, who have a shorter life span, the percentages are lower: 61 percent in non-smokers and 26 percent in smokers. Overall, smoking shortens the life of men by twelve years and that of women by eleven years. That is why we said that if you intend to live a long and healthy life, the most important recommendation we can give you is to not smoke.

Smoking, of course, is not the only assault that accelerates the aging process. In previous chapters, we have talked about obesity, which creates a state of chronic inflammation in the body that shortens life. We talked about how the human body needs to be active to stimulate its mechanisms of regeneration and repair, while a sedentary lifestyle accelerates the degradation of organs and tissues. We talked about stress, which has a direct detrimental effect because it shortens telomeres and promotes inflammation, and has an indirect effect because it leads to unhealthy behaviors. And we have talked about the protective effect of a varied diet without excess, as well as the risks of the abuse of salt, sugar, and saturated fats.

If you stop and think about it, all the unhealthy behaviors that accelerate the aging process have something in common. They all favor short-term gratification over long-term benefits. It's the immediate pleasure of sugar, tobacco, or the couch versus the abstract desire to be well tomorrow.

That is how our brain works, and that is how society operates. I want it all, and I want it now, as Freddie Mercury sang. If we take an honest look in the mirror, we must acknowledge that we are poorly equipped to resist temptation. We have brain structures that have evolved for hundreds of millions of years to respond to the call of pleasure. Conversely, we have no control center in the brain that responds to the call of health.

> If you stop and think about it, all unhealthy behaviors that accelerate the aging process have something in common. They all favor short-term gratification over long-term benefits. The immediate pleasure of sugar, tobacco, or the couch versus the abstract desire to be well tomorrow.

Do not misunderstand us. We are not saying that pleasurable experiences are negative and should be avoided. We would enjoy life very little if we gave up every form of pleasure. But if we have a minimum of expectations for the future, it is convenient to not lose sight that some of these experiences may be hurting us in the end.

In the absence of a brain structure specialized in protecting health, the best strategy we have for controlling our tendency to act in the short term is motivation. When you are motivated by something, it means having a goal that goes beyond short-term urgency and being willing to give up what you want the most at that moment to get something that matters to you later.

Caring for our health and enjoying a long life is one of the long-term objectives that, for many people, is worthwhile. It is not the ultimate goal. Every person is free to decide what his or her priorities are. But in our opinion, there are few goals that may be more important. And if you have come this far in this book, you probably agree.

Let us assume that you trust in the future, that you wish to live on this planet for many years, and that you are motivated to care for your health. What else can you do? Think about what the main causes of disease and premature death are, and you will have a response. Because these are diseases that shorten life and reduce quality of life. They are, therefore, the ones to prevent and diagnose early. To find out what they are, researchers at Harvard University in the 1990s devised a unity of measure that took into account both the years of life lost due to premature death and the years with poor quality of life. Known as the DALY (Disability Adjusted Life Years), this unit best reflects the years lived in good health and is the best guide when deciding the best prevention strategies and early diagnosis.

In developed countries, the main cause of DALY—that

is, years of health lost—are cardiovascular diseases, followed in this order by cancer, musculoskeletal pains, and diseases of the nervous system.

Within cardiovascular illnesses, the most important risk factor is hypertension, which causes nearly two million deaths per year in developed countries and more than nine million in the world. Nine million, so that you can get an idea of the magnitude of this tragedy, is triple the deaths caused by AIDS, tuberculosis, and malaria combined. And almost all of these are avoidable premature deaths.

To prevent them, the American Heart Association (AHA) recommends we begin taking our blood pressure at the age of twenty. It is performed with quick and simple test that, in Spain, is available in pharmacies. If the result is less than 120/80 millimeters of mercury, it is recommended to repeat the test every two years. If the maximum is higher than 120 or the minimum is lower than 80, it is recommended that you go to the doctor to prevent your hypertension from getting higher.

It may seem like an overreaction to start monitoring blood pressure at the age of twenty if cardiovascular diseases rarely manifest before the age of fifty. But it has the advantage of detecting the problem in its early stages, when there are more options to correct it. Especially with hypertension, which does not usually present symptoms and often goes unnoticed unless one checks it.

The AHA also recommends starting to control cholesterol and triglycerides in the bloodstream at twenty. This test is more annoying because it requires fasting before the blood analysis. But if the result is within a normal range, there is no need to repeat it for another five years.

In addition, weight control should begin around the age of twenty, according to AHA recommendations. The body mass index (BMI) should be between 18.5 and 25, for both men and women. To calculate it, two simple operations on a calculator will suffice: divide your weight (in kilos) by your height (in meters), and then divide the result by your height again.

For example, for a person who measures 1.75 meters and weighs 70 kilos, divide 70 by 1.75, which gives us 40. Then divide 40 again by 1.75, which gives us 22.9. This body mass index of 22.9 corresponds to what is called an ideal weight. If the result had been more than 25, this person would be considered overweight. If it had been more than 30, they would be considered obese, which requires medical attention. If it had been less than 18.5, they would be considered underweight, which also requires medical attention.

Finally, the AHA recommends checking your blood sugar

levels as early as the age of forty-five, and to repeat the analysis at least every three years. An excessive level may be the prelude to type 2 diabetes, which significantly increases the risk of cardiovascular disease.

If you do these checkups and take appropriate corrective measures if the results are abnormal, you can rest easy. Your risk of having a heart attack, a stroke, or any other premature accident of blood circulation will be minimal.

This leaves cancers as the next big problem that should be prevented and diagnosed early. Unfortunately, not all cancers can be avoided or detected in their early stages. God plays dice with our cells, remember? There is a lot of luck in biology. We can have bad luck, nothing more than bad luck, and we still do not have a simple test such as the analysis of cholesterol or blood pressure that can tell us if we have or will have cancer.

In the not very distant future, we will probably have this test. From a blood analysis, we could know if there is DNA circulating through the arteries because of cancer. This is called a liquid biopsy. There are dozens of research groups in the world working now to develop a test of this type. While awaiting the liquid biopsy for early diagnosis, we have specific tests to detect some of the most common cancers in time.

The most common cancer in Spain is colorectal cancer, which might surprise you because there is a lack of awareness about the frequency and the gravity of this type of cancer. A simple feces analysis starting at the age of fifty is recommended, which poses no trouble beyond collecting the sample and taking it to the clinic. In the case of hidden blood detected in the stool, a colonoscopy is required to check if there is a cancer.

For women age fifty and older, mammograms are recommended to detect breast cancer tumors before they cause symptoms, when the chances of cure are almost 100 percent. If there is a family history of breast cancer at an early age, consult a medical specialist to see if it is appropriate to do a mammogram sooner.

Another cancer that affects women is cervical cancer (or uterine cancer). It is the cause of more than 250,000 deaths a year worldwide. It can easily be counteracted with a gynecological cytology (Pap smear), that detects precancerous lesions or nascent tumors that can be treated successfully. Given that the vast majority of cervical cancers are caused by sexually transmitted papilloma virus, it is recommended to begin cytology shortly after the beginning of sexual activity. For this same reason, vaccination against papilloma virus in adolescence drastically reduces the risk of developing cervical cancer later in life. On this point, the data is clear, and there is complete agreement between medical societies.

In men, on the other hand, there is no agreement on the appropriateness of screening for prostate cancer, which is most common in the male population. The two current possible tests—rectal examination and analysis of the PSA protein in blood—have two disadvantages. First, they do not detect all cancer cases (what in medicine is called a false negative, because the result might be negative when it should be positive). Secondly, not all the suspected cases that are detected are cancer (what is called a false positive, because the result should be positive when negative). In the absence of a more precise test, the best recommendation that can be made today is to consult a urologist, starting at the sixth decade of life, to assess if it is advisable to perform a test based on risk factors and symptoms of each person.

There is no precise evidence yet that can be recommended to the entire population to pre-emptively diagnose neurodegenerative diseases such as Alzheimer's. As with prostate cancer, when in doubt, you should consult a specialist who will assess in a personalized way if it is advisable to perform an exploration.

Given this uncertainty about what the future holds, companies have emerged that promise answers based on the language of genomics. This business is not new. Before, there was palm reading or tarot cards to guess the future; today, genome analysis is available. This is useful in some cases; for example, to decide the best treatment of a cancer or the risk of developing any specific disease. But it does not predict our entire future as much as Laplace might have liked.

> Enjoying a long and lasting life depends a great deal on ourselves. It depends on whether we decide to take the reins of our own health and take responsibility in our self-care, or if, on the contrary, we prefer not to assume this responsibility.

Maybe you think we are exaggerating: "How can we compare tarot cards with genome analysis!? Tarot is not based on any rational logic, while the genome is based on a scientific method." Alright, fine. But look at what they have in common. Both are businesses taking advantage of human anxiety about the future. Both give answers that are credible but not necessarily true. Both invite us to believe what we are told, even if we do not understand it. And both refer to causes that are beyond our control to explain what happens to us. Whether things go wrong or right, it is either destiny or, the modern version, the genome. That is exactly the opposite of what we have tried to teach you in this book.

The genome, fortunately, is not fate. We do not choose the

genes we have, but what our genes do depends to some extent on decisions we make. It depends on everything we have explained in previous chapters. On our diet, our level of physical activity, our intellectual activity, how we manage our emotions...Enjoying a long and lasting life depends in great part on ourselves. It depends on whether we decide to take the reins of our health into our own hands and assume responsibility for our self-care, or if we prefer not to assume this responsibility—to give up making decisions about our own body, and to forsake being masters of our future.

Basic Prevention Measures Starting at 50

| Do not smoke | Practice physical activity | Have a healthy diet | If you drink alcohol, do so in moderation |

To prevent cardiovascular disease

Check your blood pressure at least once every 2 years

Control your cholesterol and blood sugar levels

If you have been a smoker, at age 65 check to see if you have an abdominal aortic aneurysm

To prevent cancer

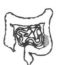

Colorectal cancer: get tested for early diagnosis after age 50

Breast cancer: mammography starting at the age of 50 every 1 to 2 years

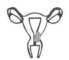

Cervical cancer: have a cytology at least once every 3 years

MENTAL HEALTH

Get a screening test for depression after age 50

OSTEOPOROSIS

Get a bone density test after age 65

IMMUNITY

Get a flu shot every autumn

Source: Adapted from the recommendations from The American Heart Association and The Centers for Disease Control and Prevention

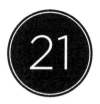

HOW LONG DO WE WANT TO LIVE?

WHAT THE WORLD WILL BE LIKE IF WE LIVE TO BE ONE HUNDRED

There will come a day when it will be normal to live more than one hundred years. It may sound utopian right now. But there was a time, four or five generations ago, which is barely a speck in human history, when a life expectancy of eighty would have seemed utopian and not normal. And if we go back a hundred generations, which remains a speck in time, it would have seemed utopian to live past sixty. And yet here we are, living the life of Methuselah. That is how we would be seen by our ancestors of the Middle Ages or the Paleolithic period. As supernatural beings who dominate incomprehensible technologies and enjoy unbelievable longevity.

Nothing like a bit of historical perspective to realize that human life tends to lengthen. And, if we consider all the progress in the biology of aging that we have explained throughout this book, it seems inevitable that one day we will overcome the symbolic barrier of one hundred years. The question is not whether it will be normal to live more than that. The question is when.

Now that we have reached this point, let me ask another question: how many of you would want to live for a hundred years? And if you could live longer, who would want to live two hundred years? Or five hundred. Where do we draw the line? How do you feel about the power to live a thousand years? Would you like to be immortal?

It is not going to be possible; do not panic. Human beings are perishable by nature. Science will not make you immortal or give a two-hundred-year lifespan to anyone of our generation.

But it is a good exercise, because it forces us to consider how long we would like to extend our lifespan. A hundred years? Okay, I am in. Two hundred? Ugh, no way.

But, why is one hundred plausible and two hundred not? Where is the limit between what is acceptable and what is not? When looking for a response, we realize that the important question is not whether we want to live longer, but how we want to live that extended life.

So, allow us to ask you how. The first answer that tends to come to mind, or at least the one given to us by most people who were asked the question, is good health. If we live longer, may it be to enjoy life and not to suffer. It makes no sense that medicine strives to prolong life if we are disabled, sick, lonely, and sad.

But, as we have explained in previous chapters, the longer we live, the less time we spend being sick. You can revisit the graph in chapter 7: in the United States, the general population spends an average of fifteen years in poor health; in people who are older than ninety, that time is reduced to nine years; and in supercentenarians, it is only five years.

Therefore, when it becomes the norm to live over a hundred years, it will also become the norm to have great health up to a very advanced age. Because it will only be possible to live so many years if the major causes of premature illnesses that today punish the majority of the population have been reduced.

Then, we ask how. Assuming that you will have acceptable health, would you want to live beyond one hundred? Up to 122 years, like Jeanne Calment, or even longer? You see, it is not an easy question. You can reply quickly and spontaneously, and say yes or no. Both replies are valid; there is no right or wrong answer. But try to explain why.

> Beyond health is fulfillment. It is only worth living longer if living longer is worth it. This is going to be the big challenge when the science of aging has achieved the goal of extending life.

The explanation tends to be that beyond health, there is fulfillment. It is only worth living longer if living longer is worth it. This is going to be the big challenge when the science of aging has achieved the goal of extending life.

It is not a very original idea, by the way. Abraham Lincoln is said to have uttered it 150 years ago: "In the end, it's not the years in your life that count. It's the life in your years." Or Pliny the Elder in the first century: "Nature has given men no better thing than shortness of life." There are many ways of expressing this, and many writers and speakers have done it.

If you allow us to make a prediction, we suspect that to achieve fulfillment in advanced ages will be more difficult than achieving health. The first difficulty we can anticipate is in demographics. A society where it is usual to live more than one hundred years will inevitably be a society with few children and young people.

If you do not like being with children, this may seem like good news. But bear in mind that, for many people, family is a source of eudaimonic wellbeing. It is something that gives meaning to life, as mentioned in chapter 10. Taking care of children and watching them grow is often a source of stress, but also of joy, and for most mothers and fathers, it is something worth living for.

> We are moving towards a future in which science and medicine may prolong life, but we run the risk of depriving the elderly of reasons that give meaning to their lives. If anyone has any ideas to address this problem, they are welcome to share. It's not going to be an easy problem to solve.

In addition, young people in all societies bring new ideas, new illusions, and new ways to see and change the world. They bring creativity, innovation, and renewed enthusiasm. New blood, as the saying goes. A change in the demographic structure, with more people of advanced age and fewer young people, will most likely turn dynamic societies into more conservative ones. This does not have to be negative. It will depend on how each community adapts to their new reality. But it will have important political, economic, and social consequences.

Another difficulty is that people over eighty are almost all retired. The way the economy is currently regulated, increasing life expectancy from eighty to one hundred does not prolong the years of professional activity but that of retirement. And professional activity is not only essential to personal autonomy but also, along with family, a second great source of eudaimonic satisfaction. It is not for everyone, certainly, but it is for those who intend to contribute to society with their work. In Japan, the country with the highest life expectancy in the world, 80 percent of the elderly would like to continue working beyond the retirement age and contribute to the economy instead of relying on aid.

We are moving, therefore, towards a future in which science and medicine may extend life, but we run the risk of depriving the elderly of reasons that give meaning to their lives. If anyone has any ideas how to address this problem, they are welcome to share. It is not going to be an easy problem to solve.

The demographic issue can be minimized by widening the gap between generations. It is something that we have already begun to do without meaning to. A few decades ago in Spain, it was normal to have children between the ages of twenty and thirty, and grandchildren around fifty. Today, people rarely have children before thirty, or grandchildren before sixty.

But while the average life expectancy of the population has increased, the age limit on fertility has remained constant, with a border that is below fifty for most women. It is somewhat surprising because death seems to be a more difficult enemy than infertility, but we have advanced further in extending life than in extending the period in which women can have children. Therefore, we cannot expect to increase the age of reproduction at the same pace that longevity increases. It will be difficult to sustain the eudaimonic wellbeing in our advanced age if we follow this path. Can we hold on to it by extending the years of professional activity? It is also going to be difficult. I am sure many of you don't think this is a very good idea. If work is not fulfilling, working more years will not fulfill you, either. However, if you are one of those who prefer to continue working instead of retiring, and are able to contribute to society and not be a hindrance, then staying active is as beneficial for you as it is for the others. But in Spain and other European countries, this is not possible. One can be retired despite being in full form and eager to continue. Either way, even if retirement is recognized as a right and not an obligation, for many people it will not be enough to have a good quality of life with eudaimonic wellbeing at an advanced age. Because they first need to like the work they do, which is not always the case.

Which leads us to an unprecedented situation in the history of mankind. For all the research to delay aging to make sense, we must decide what we want to do when we get older. We are talking about centenarians and super-centenarians. Older than any previous generation.

We cannot give you an answer. We do not have it, and the answer may vary according to each person. For some, the answer may be in religion, where they find fulfillment and meaning to their existence. For others, as we have stated in previous chapters, it may be in looking for a way to contribute to the community after retirement. We may not want to continue working on the same thing we have done for the last thirty or forty years, which is understandable. But surely we can find other ways to help others and feel useful. This is, for example, exactly what the man we talked about in chapter 10 did; after losing his position as museum director, he dedicated his life to deactivating war mines.

Then there is the Pei solution, the architect we talked about in chapter 11, who continues working on projects at ninety-nine years of age because he finds the inner motivation to continue to learn and not be a slave to social stereotypes.

We have already told you that we do not have the answer. But in our experience and what we have learned from people like those we have introduced throughout this book, who find meaning in a long life and continue to be motivated well into their advanced age, they tend to be people who have a sense of transcendence. A feeling that life does not end with death. That they have planted the seeds for their future and have left a footprint on the world. They are people seeking longevity who accept their mortality.

The seeds they plant may be biological, in DNA form that they have bequeathed to their children and grandchildren. But many times, those seeds are cultural. They are the ideas and values they have passed on, the example they have given, everything that has been done, and what has been taught to them. This book is an example of that. It is a small bag of seeds. You can accept or reject the ideas that we have proposed. You can transform them and make them your own. You can combine them with other ideas and create something completely new—something that has never been created by anyone else. If you prefer, you can forget about it. Or share them with others, who might modify them and, in turn, pass them on to future generations.

How to Delay Aging: The Integral Vision

The choices we make as individuals and as a community affect processes that occur in our cells in a way that allows the delay of the aging process

SCALE

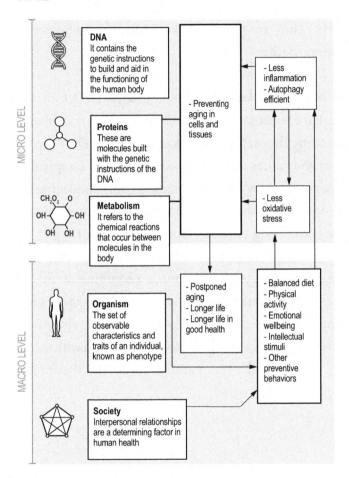

TWENTY BASIC TIPS FOR ENJOYING A LONG LIFE

TIP 1

PURPOSE: QUALITY OF LIFE

Remember that the purpose of taking care of yourself isn't living many years— it's living them in good health.

CHAPTER 1

TIP 2

DON'T SUCCUMB TO YOUR AGE BIAS

Our age says little about ourselves. It's just a number; it doesn't make us who we are. Don't allow people to judge you because of your age, and don't judge others by the same token.

CHAPTER 1

TIP 3

DON'T WAIT UNTIL YOU'RE SICK TO START TAKING CARE OF YOURSELF

Your health is a long-term investment. What we do throughout our life can speed up aging or slow it down.

CHAPTERS 6 & 8

TIP 4

THINK GLOBAL, ACT LOCAL

Aging is what we experience in our entire body at the macroscopic level, as a reflection of what is happening on a microscopic level, in our cells and tissues. Fortunately, we can modify what happens in our cells and tissues with the actions we take and the decisions we make.

CHAPTERS 3 TO 8

TIP 5

AVOID AGGRESSIONS THAT ACCELERATE AGING

A sedentary lifestyle, smoking, obesity, and stress are aggressions that damage our cells, speeding up the deterioration of human body tissue.

CHAPTERS 6 & 20

TIP 6

REMEMBER THAT AGING CAN BE SLOWED DOWN WITH AN ACTIVE LIFESTYLE

Keeping active at the physical, social, and intellectual levels favors biochemical processes in the cells that help maintain good health.

CHAPTER 12

TIP 7

ESTABLISH A BALANCED DIET, BOTH IN TERMS OF QUALITY AND QUANTITY

Both excessive and deficient eating habits cause damage. Try to keep your diet varied and vegetable-rich, and avoid eating too much red meat and processed foods.

CHAPTER 17

TIP 8

TO KEEP YOUR BRAIN IN GOOD SHAPE, KEEP FIT

Physical activity slows down cognitive decline. A sedentary lifestyle speeds it up.

CHAPTER 14

TIP 9

DON'T MISTAKE PHYSICAL ACTIVITY FOR SPORT

Playing sports is a good way to remain physically active, but it's not the only way. Walking at a rapid pace, taking the stairs rather than the elevator, or tending to your garden are equally healthy physical activities.

CHAPTER 13

TIP 10

COMBINE DIFFERENT TYPES OF EXERCISE

Physical activity is like your diet—it should be varied. Combine various aerobic activities for your cardio-respiratory health, resistance activities for your muscles, and coordination and balance activities to improve your control over your body's movements.

CHAPTER 13

TIP 11

MAKE YOUR MUSCLES WORK

Remember that your muscles aren't passive tissues that only provide brute force; by exercising them, the necessary molecules are segregated and provide a well-functioning human body. Good musculoskeletal health will also help you prevent pain in the neck, back, hips, or knees, improving your quality of life.

CHAPTERS 6 & 13

TIP 12

MAKE YOUR BRAIN WORK

Maintaining your mental activity slows down the deterioration of cognitive capabilities and, in the specific case of people with Alzheimer's, delays the onset of symptoms. Speaking multiple languages or playing a musical instrument have a protective effect on the brain.

CHAPTER 14

TIP 13
DON'T ISOLATE YOURSELF

Don't neglect your emotional relationships. Being in touch with other people, be they family, friends, or colleagues, helps maintain good emotional health, boosting longevity and quality of life.

CHAPTER 15

TIP 14
FIND YOUR INTERNAL MOTIVATION

On the Japanese island of Okinawa, they call this ikigai. It's the purpose each person finds in their life, the reason to get out of bed each morning. It's something personal and non-transferable, which means that every person has to discover it for themselves. When we find it, we obtain greater control over our lives; we depend less on what other people think or expect of us, and we boast lower stress levels and higher levels of wellbeing.

CHAPTERS 8, 10 & 11

TIP 15

DON'T GIVE UP ON BEING ACTIVE WHEN YOU RETIRE

Retirement usually comes at an age when people are healthy and able to continue contributing to the community. To enjoy the stage of life starting with retirement, look for gratifying activities rather than being inactive.

CHAPTERS 11 & 21

TIP 16

DON'T GIVE UP ON YOUR SEXUALITY

Don't succumb to social stereotypes. Interest in sex, while not universal, is normal in older adults.

CHAPTER 16

TIP 17

DON'T FALL FOR MIRACLE CURES

Right now, there's no pill, potion, cream, or dietary supplement that can guarantee rejuvenating effects. There will probably be such options in the future, but first they'll have to show their efficacy and safety.

CHAPTER 19

TIP 18

DON'T FORGET ABOUT MEDICAL CHECKUPS

Doing the basic checkups recommended by doctors' associations—including controlling blood pressure and cholesterol levels, to name a few—is essential for an early diagnosis of problems and preventing complications.

CHAPTER 20

TIP 19

HAVE TRUST IN THE FUTURE

For the majority of the population, wellbeing increases after turning fifty. If you don't neglect your health, you'll probably enjoy a long life with a considerable quality of life.

CHAPTER 10

TIP 20

FINAL MESSAGE

Aging can't be undone, but it can be slowed down.

ADDITIONAL READING FOR A LONG LIFE

CHAPTER 1: AGE IS JUST A NUMBER

Attitudes **towards the chronological age** studied in Alter, A., and H. E. Hershfield, "People Search for Meaning When They Approach a New Decade in Chronological Age," *PNAS* vol. 111, no. 48, (2014): pp. 17066-17070.

The Duke University study on the **calculation of biological age** described in Belsky, D. W., et al., "Quantification of Biological Aging in Young Adults," *PNAS* vol. 112, no. 309, (2014): pp. 4104-4110.

The **formula to calculate the biological age of the heart** is available at www.cdc.gov/heartdisease/heartage.html

The article from *Wall Street Journal* from which part of the chart data was extracted is "Why Everything You Know about Aging Is Probably Wrong," Anne Tergesen, published December 2, 2014.

CHAPTER 2: WRINKLES

The **Borges reference to mirrors** appears in the initial paragraph of "Tlön, Uqbar, Orbis Tertius," the story that opens the volume *Ficciones*, Alianza Editorial, Madrid, 2002.

The clinical description of the **smoker face model** is found in Model, D., "Smoker's Face: An Underrated Clinical Sign?" *British Medical Journal* vol. 291, no. 6511, (1985): pp. 1760-1762.

For a broader view of the **effects of tobacco on the skin**, see Ortiz, A., and Grando, S. A., "Smoking and the Skin," *International Journal of Dermatology* vol. 51, no. 3, (2012): pp. 250-262.

The **effects of solar radiation on the skin** are described in Helfrich, Y. R., et al., "Overview of Aging Skin and Photoaging," *Dermatology Nursing* vol. 20, no. 3, (2008): pp. 177-183.

To understand human skin, not only from a medical and biological point of view, but also aesthetic and cultural, we recommend the book *Skin, a Natural History* by Nina Jablonski, University of California Press, 2006.

CHAPTER 3: CELLS NEVER SLEEP

The improvement of **crystallized intelligence** with age is explained in Hartshorne, J. K., and L. Germine, "When Does Cognitive Functioning Peak? The Asynchronous Rise and Fall of Different Cognitive Abilities across the Lifespan," *Psychological Science* vol. 26, no. 4, (2005): pp. 433-443.

A systematic review of **cellular changes** associated with aging is found in López-Otin, C., et al., "The Hallmarks of Aging" *Cell* vol. 153, no. 6, (2013): pp. 1194-1217.

For a review of the research on **sirtuins and its relationship with aging**: Guarente, L., "Calorie Restriction and Sirtuins Revisited," *Genes and Development* vol. 27, no. 19, (2013): pp. 2072-2085.

For a specific analysis of the **potential of sirtuins to prevent cardiovascular deterioration**: Winnik, S., et al., "Protective Effects of Sirtuins in Cardiovascular Diseases: From Bench to Bedside," *European Heart Journal* vol. 36, no. 48, (2005): pp. 3404-3412.

For a review of the relationship between **telomeres** and aging: Blackburn. E., et al., "Human Telomere Biology: A Contributory and Interactive Factor in Aging, Disease Risks and Protection," *Science* vol. 350, no. 6265, (2015): pp. 1193-1198.

CHAPTER 4: RENEW OR DIE

The importance of **fibrosis** in the pathologies associated with age is explained in Rockey, D. C., et al., "Fibrosis—A Common Pathway to Organ Injury and Failure," *New England Journal of Medicine* vol. 373, no. 1, (2015): pp. 1138-1149.

For a review of the relationship of **autophagy** with sickness associated with age, see Glick, D., et al., "Autophagy: Cellular and Molecular Mechanisms," *Journal of Pathology* vol. 221, no. 1, (2010): pp. 3-12.

For the **influence of stem cells on aging** see Goodell, M. A., and Rando, T. A., "Stem Cells and Healthy Aging," *Science* vol. 350, no. 6265, (2015): pp. 1199-1204.

A strategy to **maintain the role of stem cells** and prevent deterioration of the tissues is discussed in detail in Geiger, H., "Depleting Senescent Cells to Combat Aging," *Nature Medicine* vol. 22, no. 1, (2016): pp. 23-24.

CHAPTER 5: THE ARROW OF TIME

A brief and excellent explanation of why the **passage of time** is a thermodynamic effect is found in the sixth chapter of the book *Sette brevi lezioni di fisica*, by Carlo Rovelli, Adelphi, 2014.

CHAPTER 6: EXPIRATION DATE

This first major study identifying that **hand strength predicts the state of health** in subsequent years is Rantanen, T., et al., "Midlife Hand Grip Strength as a Predictor of Old Age Disability," *JAMA* vol. 281, no. 6, (1999): pp. 558-560.

The larger study on grip strength: Leong, D. P., et al., "Prognostic Value of Grip Strength: Findings from the Prospective Urban Rural Epidemiology (PURE) Study," *The Lancet* vol. 386, no. 990, (2015): pp. 266-273.

The **relationship between walking speed and the risk of death** in the following years is explored in Elbaz, A., et al., "Association of Walking Speed in Late Midlife with Mortality: Results from the Whitehall II Cohort Study," *Age* vol. 35, no. 3, (2013): pp. 943-952.

A recent review of the **relationship between the walking speed and their state of health** is found in Middleton, A., et al., "Walking Speed: The Functional Vital Sign," *Journal of Aging and Physical Activity* vol. 23, no. 2, (2015): pp. 314-322.

The effects of **aging on the cardiovascular system** are described in the review article Paneni, F., et al., "The Aging Cardiovascular System: Understanding the Cellular and Clinical Level," *Journal of American College of Cardiology* vol. 69, no. 15, (2017): pp 1952-1967.

The **decline of the functional capacity** of people as they age, and how health systems should adapt, discussed in Beard, J. R., et al., "The World Report on Aging and Health: Policy Framework for Healthy Aging," *The Lancet* vol. 387, no. 10033, (2016): pp. 2145-2154.

CHAPTER 7: SECRETS OF THE CENTENARIANS

The results of the Study of Centenarians of New England on the **influence of genetics in cases of extreme longevity** presented in Sebastiani, P., et al., "Genetic Signatures of Exceptional Longevity in Humans," *PLoS One* vol. 7, no. 1, (2012): e29848. doi: 10.1371/journal. pone.0029848.

A **meta-analysis** that synthesizes the data of various studies: Sebastiani, P., et al., "Meta-analysis of Genetic Variants Associated with Human Exceptional Longevity," *Aging* vol. 5, no. 9, (2013): pp. 653-661.

The influence of the **FOXO3A gene** on extreme longevity is identified in Willcox B. J., et al., "FOXO3A Genotype is Strongly Associated with Human Longevity," *PNAS*, vol. 105, no. 37, (2008): pp. 13987-13992.

The influence of **other genes** explored in Fortney, K., et al. "Genome-wide Scan Informed by Age-related Disease Identifies Loci for Exceptional Human Longevity," *PLoS Genetics* vol. 11, no. 12, (2015): e1005728. doi: 10.1371/journal.pgen.1005728.

The observation that **people who live long lives have good health until very advanced ages**, derived from the New England Study of Centenarians, in Andersen, S. L., et al., "Health Span Approximates Life Span Among Many Supercentenarians: Compression of Morbidity at the Approximate Limit of Life Span," *Journals of Gerontology Series A: Biological Sciences and Medical Sciences* vol. 67, no. 4, (2012): pp. 395-405.

The **biological limit** of human longevity in Dong, X., et al., "Evidence for a Limit to Human Lifespan," *Nature* vol. 538, no. 7624, (2016): pp. 257-259 doi: 10.1038/nature19793.

CHAPTER 8: THE BLUE ZONES

The original article that **identified the blue zone of Barbagia in Sardinia** is found in Poulain, M., et al., "Identification of a Geographic Area Characterized by Extreme Longevity in the Sardinia Island: the AKEA Study," *Experimental Gerontology* vol. 39, no. 9, (2004): pp. 1423-1429.

The **Centenarians of Okinawa study**, begun in 1975, has been presented in more than two hundred scientific articles and can be accessed from www.okicent.org/publications.html The most important aspects of the study are detailed in Wilcox, D. C., et al., "They Really Are That Old: A Validation Study of Prevalence Okinawa Centenarian Study," *Journals of Gerontology Series A: Biological Sciences and Medical Sciences* vol. 63, no. 4, (2008): pp. 338-349.

You can access articles from scientific studies of **Adventist** Health at University of Loma Linda website: http://publichealth.llu.edu/adventist-health-studies/scientific-publications They focus mainly on the influence of environmental factors—primarily the diet—on morbidity and mortality.

Dan Buettner describes his research on the blue areas in the book *The Blue Zones*, National Geographic Society, 2012.

The study concluding that male **sexual orientation is associated with a gene** located in the X chromosome is found in Hamer, D. H., et al., "A Linkage Between DNA Markers on the X Chromosome and Male Sexual Orientation," *Science* vol. 261, no. 5119, (1993): pp. 321-327.

CHAPTER 9: WHY WOMEN LIVE LONGER

The study on the **longevity of the eunuchs** of the Chosun dynasty of Korea is in Min, K. J., et al., "The Lifespan of Korean Eunuchs," *Current Biology* vol. 22, no. 18, (2012): pp. 792-793.

A review of the mechanisms by which **estrogen** may regulate longevity is found in Dulken, B., and A. Brunet, "Stem Cell Aging and Sex: Are We Missing Something?" *Cell Stem Cell* vol. 16, no. 6, (2015): pp. 588-590.

The research on the **loss of the regenerative ability of the muscles** with age conducted by the Universitat Pompeu Fabra of Barcelona, is in Sousa-Victor, P., et al., "Geriatric Muscle Stem Cells Switch Reversible Quiescence into Senescence," *Nature* vol. 506, no. 7488, (2014): pp. 316-321.

The baseline study on risks and benefits of **hormone** therapy in women is Rossouw, J. E., et al., "Risks and Benefits of Estrogen plus Progestin in Healthy Postmenopausal Women: Principal Results from the Women's Health Initiative Randomized Controlled Trial," *JAMA* vol. 288, no. 3, (2002): pp. 321-333.

CHAPTER 10: THE CURVE OF HAPPINESS

The evolution of the **three different types of wellbeing (hedonic, evaluative, and eudaimonic)** throughout life in different countries is analyzed in Steptoe, A., et al., "Subjective Wellbeing, Health and Aging," *The Lancet* vol. 385, no. 9968, (2015): pp. 640-648.

The study that establishes the **relationship between eudaimonic wellness and the reduction of risk of stress** is Yu, L., et al., "Purpose in Life and Cerebral Infarcts in Community-Dwelling Older People," *Stroke* vol. 46, no. 4, (2015): pp. 1071-1076.

The details of the **ELSA study** done in England are described in Steptoe, A., et al., "Cohort Profile: the English Longitudinal Study of Ageing," *International Journal of Epidemiology* vol. 42, no. 6, (2013): pp. 1640-1648.

The classic look of **the seven ages** of life was expressed by Shakespeare in one of his famous poems, the monologue "All the world is a stage," recited by the character Jacques in the comedy *As You Like It*.

CHAPTER 11: FROM PYRAMIDS TO SKYSCRAPERS

The **poem by William B. Yeats** about the passage of time that begins with "That is no country for old men" is "Sailing to Byzantium," from the volume *The Tower*, published in 1928.

The **rise of hope among older people** is found in Mathers, C. D., et al. "Causes of International Increase in Older Age Life Expectancy," *The Lancet* vol. 385, no. 9967, (2015): pp. 540-548.

The **impact of the increase of survival on the quality of life** in older populations is analyzed comprehensively in the macro study: GBD 2013 DALYs and HALE Collaborators "Global, Regional and National Disability-adjusted Life-years (DALYs) for 306 Diseases and Injuries and Healthy Life Expectancy (HALE) for 188 Countries, 1990-2013: Quantifying the Epidemiological Transition," *The Lancet*, vol. 386, no. 10009, (2015): pp. 2145-2191.

An analysis on the **macroeconomic implications of the age increase of the population** is in Bloom, D. E., et al., "Macroeconomic Implications of Population Ageing and Selected Policy Responses," *The Lancet* vol. 385, no. 9968, (2015): pp. 649-657.

CHAPTER 12: THE TREE OF LIFE

The **essential book on fractals** by Mandelbrot, B., *The Fractal Geometry of Nature*, Ed. W. H. Freeman and Co. Existe traducción española: *La geometría fractal de la naturaleza*, Ed. Tusquets, Barcelona, 1997. However, its seven hundred pages may discourage those who simply wish to familiarize themselves with the subject.

For a more accessible introduction, we recommend: Mandelbrot, B., *Los objetos fractales*, Ed. Tusquets, Barcelona, 1987.

CHAPTER 13: NEVER TOO LATE FOR HEALTHY WORKOUTS

The **relationship between the metabolism and aging** is analyzed in Finkel, T., "The Metabolic Regulation of Aging," vol. 21, no. 12, (2015): pp. 1416-1423.

Another excellent introduction is found in Bitto, A., et al., "Biochemical Genetic Pathways that Modulate Aging in Multiple Species," *Cold Spring Harbor Perspectives in Medicine* vol. 5, no. 11, (2015): pp. 25-49. This article is part of the book *Aging: The Longevity Dividend*, edited by Jay Olshansky, George Martin, and James Kirkland, Cold Spring Harbor Laboratory Press, 2016.

The **metabolic effects of physical activity on the muscle tissue** is described in Egan, B., et al., "Exercise Metabolism and the Molecular Regulation of Skeletal Muscle Adaptation," *Cell Metabolism* vol. 17, no. 2, (2013): pp. 162-184.

The study that indicates that **practicing physical activity a few days a week is healthier than exercising every day** is Armstrong, M., et al., "Frequent Physical Activity May Not Reduce Vascular Disease Risk as Much as Moderate Activity," *Circulation* vol. 131, no. 8, (2015): pp. 721-729.

The research that revealed that the **telomeres of people who are physically active** are longer than those who are sedentary is Werner, C., et al., "Physical Exercise Prevents Cellular Senescence in Circulating Leukocytes and in the Vessel Wall," *Circulation* vol. 120, no. 24, (2009): pp. 2438-2447.

CHAPTER 14: BRAIN FITNESS

The study that evaluated **how the different cognitive faculties vary in age** is from Hartshorne, J., and Germine, L., "When Does Cognitive Functioning Peak? The Asynchronous Rise and Fall of Different Cognitive Abilities Across the Life Span," *Psychological Science* vol. 26, no. 4, (2015): pp. 433-443.

An exhaustive revision on **the relationship between intellectual faculties and aging** can be found in Lindenberger, U., "Human Cognitive Aging: Corriger la Fortune?" *Science* vol. 346, no. 6209, (2014): pp. 572-578.

The influence of **musical education to prevent cognitive decline** at advanced ages, among other studies, in Gooding, L. F., et al., "Musical Training and Late-life Cognition," *American Journal of Alzheimer's Disease and Other Dementias* vol. 29, no. 4, (2014): pp. 333-343.

Multiple studies have analyzed the **relationship between physical activity and cognitive decline**, as well as the influence of physical activity to prevent the deterioration of intellectual capacities. An excellent summary is found in Hillman. C. H., et al., "Be Smart, Exercise Your Heart: Exercise Effects on Brain and Cognition," *Nature Reviews Neuroscience* vol. 9, no. 1, (2008): pp. 58-65.

A **synthesis of the study results** on the relationship between physical activity and cognitive deterioration is found in Sofi, F., et al., "Physical Activity and Risk of Cognitive Decline: A Meta-Analysis of Prospective Studies," *Journal of Internal Medicine* vol. 269, no. 1, (2011): pp. 107-117.

The study at King's College of London that establishes a **correlation between cognitive abilities and muscle strength** is Steves, C. J., et al., "Kicking Back Cognitive Ageing: Leg Power Predicts Cognitive Ageing after Ten Years in Older Female Twins," *Gerontology* vol. 62, no. 2, (2016): pp. 138-149.

The **relationship between cardiovascular health and cognitive abilities in older people** was unequivocally proven in the Finger study conducted in Finland: Ngandu, T., et al., "A 2 Year Multidomain Intervention of Diet, Exercise, Cognitive Training, and Vascular Risk Monitoring Versus Control to Prevent Cognitive Decline in At-risk Elderly People (FINGER): a Randomised Controlled Trial," *The Lancet* vol. 385, no. 9984, (2015): pp. 2255-2263.

The study conducted on **middle-aged adults** to establish the relationship between cardiorespiratory health and cognitive function is: Zhu, N., et al., "Cardiorespiratory Fitness and Cognitive Function in Middle Age," The CARDIA Study vol. 82, no. 15, (2014): pp. 1339-1346.

CHAPTER 15: KEEP ON SMILING

The investigation by Elizabeth Blackburn that shows that **persistent stress shortens telomeres** is Epel, E. S., et al., "Accelerated Telomere Shortening in Response to Life Stress," *PNAS* vol. 101, no. 49, (2014): pp 17312-17315.

The **relationship between stress and inflammation** is explored in Heidt, T., et al., "Chronic Stress Activates Variable Hematopoietic Stem Cells," *Nature Medicine* vol. 20, no. 7, (2014): pp. 754-758. Other prominent studies that have addressed the question are these: Cohen, S., et al., "Chronic Stress, Glucocorticoid Receptor Resistance, Inflammation, and Disease Risk," *PNAS* vol. 109, no. 16, (2012): pp 5995-5999; Powell, N. D., et al., "Social Stress Up-Regulates Inflammatory Gene Expression in the Leukocyte Transcriptome Via ß-adrenergic Induction of Myelopoiesis," *PNAS* vol. 110, no. 41, (2013): pp. 16574-16579.

A summary of the **benefits of physical activity on emotional health in older people** is presented in the review article of Windle, G., et al., "Is Exercise Effective in Promoting Mental Well-being in Older Age? A Systematic Review," *Aging and Mental Health* vol. 14, no. 6, (2010): pp. 652-669.

The benefits of social activity on emotional health, also in older people, are discussed in Morrow-Howell, N., et al., "Effects of Volunteering on the Well-being of Older Adults," *Journal of Gerontology* vol. 58B, no. 3, (2003): pp. 137-145.

CHAPTER 16: SEX HAS NO AGE

The study that analyzed **how the interest in sex evolves in men of advanced ages** is in the Helgason, A., et al., "Sexual Desire, Erection, Orgasm and Ejaculatory Functions and Their Importance to Elderly Swedish Men: A Population Based Study," *Age and Ageing* vol. 25, no. 4, (1996): pp. 285-291.

The **evolution of sexual activity from the age of fifty and beyond eighty** in the US population is analyzed in Schick, V., et al., "Sexual Behaviors, Condom Use, and Sexual Health of Americans Over 50: Implications for Sexual Health Promotion for Older Adults," *The Journal of Sexual Medicine* vol. 7, no. 5, (2010): pp. 315-329.

The **risk factors of erectile dysfunction** have been identified in Bacon, C. G., et al., "A Prospective Study of Risk Factors for Erectile Dysfunction," *The Journal of Urology* vol. 176, no. 1, (2006): pp. 217-221. And also Selvin, E., et al., "Prevalence and Risk Factors for Erectile Dysfunction in the US," *The American Journal of Medicine* vol. 120, no. 2, (2007): pp. 151-157.

The measures of **prevention of erectile dysfunction** are summarized in the review article of Gupta, B. P., et al., "The Effect of Lifestyle Modification and Cardiovascular Risk Factor Reduction on Erectile Dysfunction," *Archives of Internal Medicine* vol. 171, no. 20, (2011): pp. 1797-1803.

The influence of **dietary flavonoids to prevent erectile dysfunction** has been analyzed in Cassidy, A., et al. "Dietary Flavonoid Intake and Incidence of Erectile Dysfunction," *American Journal of Clinical Nutrition* vol. 103, no. 2, (2016): pp. 534-541.

The most recent data on treatment with **testosterone supplements** was presented in Snyder, P. J., et al., "Effects of Testosterone Treatment in Older Men," *The New England Journal of Medicine* vol. 374, no. 7, (2016): pp. 611-624.

CHAPTER 17: EAT WELL, LIVE LONGER

The complex **relationship between diet and longevity** is summarized in the review article of Fontana, L., and Partridge, L., "Promoting Health and Longevity Through Diet: From Model Organisms to Humans," *Cell* vol. 161, no. 1, (2015): pp. 106-118.

The possibility of **a diet that provides the benefits of caloric restriction, but avoids the risk of malnutrition** is explored in Brandhorst, S., et al., "A Periodic Diet that Mimics Fasting Promotes Multi-System Regeneration, Enhanced Cognitive Performance, and Healthspan," *Cell Metabolism* vol. 22, no. 1, (2015): pp. 86-99.

The results of the study that analyzed the **effects of the Mediterranean diet on cardiovascular health** was presented in Estruch, R., et al., "Primary Prevention of Cardiovascular Disease with a Mediterranean Diet Supplemented with Extra-Virgin Olive Oil or Nuts," *The New England Journal of Medicine* vol. 378, no. 25, (2018): pp. e34.

The benefits of the **Mediterranean diet for the prevention of cognitive decline** is described in Valls-Pedret, C., et al., "Mediterranean Diet and Age-Related Cognitive Decline: Randomized Clinical Trial," *JAMA Internal Medicine* vol. 175, no. 7, (2015): pp. 1094-1103.

The **specific benefits of dried fruit** are described in Bao, Y., et al., "Association of Nut Consumption with Total and Cause-Specific Mortality," *The New England Journal of Medicine* vol. 369, no. 21, (2013): pp. 2001-2011.

The benefits of **whole grains** compared to refined in populations that do not consume a Mediterranean diet are summarized in the review article of Aune, D., et al., "Whole Grain Consumption and Risk of Cardiovascular Disease, Cancer, and All Cause and Cause Specific Mortality: Systematic Review and Dose-Response Meta-Analysis of Prospective Studies," *British Medical Journal* vol. 14, no. 353: i2716, (2016). doi: 10.1136/bmj.i2716.

The potential benefits of the **diet for the prevention of Alzheimer's** discussed in the review article of Swaminathan, A., and Jicha, G. A., "Nutrition and Prevention of Alzheimer's Dementia," *Frontiers in Aging Neuroscience* vol. 6, no. 282, (2014): p. 282.

CHAPTER 18: ANTIOXIDANTS AND FREE RADICALS

A review of the **relationship between oxidation and longevity** is Wang, Y., and Hekimi, S., "Mitochondrial Dysfunction and Longevity in Animals: Untangling the Knot," *Science* vol. 350, no. 6265, (2015): pp. 1204-1207.

The **mechanisms by which antioxidants and free radicals influence longevity** are explored in Bitto, A., et al., "Biochemical Genetic Pathways that Modulate Aging in Multiple Species," *Cold Spring Harbor Perspectives in Medicine* vol. 5, no. 11, (2015): pp. 25-49. The **central role of the mitochondria in the regulation of longevity** has been demonstrated in the National Cardiovascular Research: LaTorre-Pellicer, A., et al., (2016), "Mitochondrial and Nuclear DNA Matching Shapes and Metabolism Healthy Ageing," *Nature* vol. 535, no: 7613, (2016): pp. 561-565.

The study that found that **vitamin E does not reduce the risk of lung cancer** is The Alpha-Tocopherol, Beta Carotene Cancer Prevention Study Group, "The Effect of Vitamin E and Beta Carotene on the Incidence of Lung Cancer and Other Cancers in Male Smokers," *The New England Journal of Medicine* vol. 330, no. 15, (1994): pp. 1029-1035.

The **possible beneficial** effect of **vitamin C on the risk of lung cancer** is exposed in the meta-analysis of Luo, J., et al., "Association between Vitamin C Intake and Lung Cancer: A Dose-Response Meta-Analysis," *Scientific Reports* vol. 4, no. 6161, (2014).

CHAPTER 19: YOUTH PILLS

An extensive review of the **current research to develop drugs against the aging process** is found in Scott, C. T., and DeFrancesco, L., "Selling Long Life," *Nature Biotechnology* vol. 33, no. 1, (2015): pp. 31-40.

A further review is Riera, C. E., and Dillin, A., "Can Aging Be 'Drugged'?" *Nature Medicine* vol. 21, no. 12, (2015): pp. 1400–1405.

A detailed explanation of the **potential of the drug rapamycin** against the aging process is from Lamming, D. W., "Inhibition of the Mechanistic Target of Rapamycin (mTOR)—Rapamycin and Beyond," *Cold Spring Harbor Perspectives in Medicine* vol. 6, no 5, (2016).

The study showed that rapamycin **extends life in mice** even when they begin to get older, from Harrison, D. E., et al., "Rapamycin Fed Late in Life Extends Lifespan in Genetically Heterogeneous Mice," *Nature* vol. 460, no. 7253, (2009): pp. 392–395.

The potential of **metformin** against aging is explained in Novelle, M. G., et al. "Metformin: Hopeful Promise in the Aging Research," *Cold Spring Harbor Perspectives in Medicine* vol. 6, no. 3, (2016).

A presentation of the **study explained in TAME** Barzilai, N., et al., "Metformin as a Tool to Target Aging," *Cell Metabolism* vol. 23, no. 6, (2016): pp. 1060–1065. A summary is in Hayden, E.C., "Ageing Pushed as Treatable Condition," *Nature* vol. 522, no. 7556, (2015), pp. 265–266.

The study that has identified a **higher survival rate in people with diabetes who take metformin** than in the rest of the population is Bannister, C. A., et al., "Can People with Type 2 Diabetes Live Longer Than Those Without? A Comparison of Mortality in People Initiated with Metformin or Sulphonylurea Monotherapy and Matched, Non-diabetic Controls," *Diabetes, Obesity and Metabolism* (2014), vol. 16 (11), pp. 1165-1173.

The **potential of sirtuins to develop drugs against aging,** beyond resveratrol, is analyzed in the review article of Guarente, L., "Calorie Restriction and Sirtuins Revisited," *Genes and Development* vol. 27, no. 19, (2013): pp. 2072-2085.

In the specific field of **cardiovascular aging,** the potential of sirtuins in Winnik, S., et al., "Protective Effects of Sirtuins in Cardiovascular Diseases: From Bench to Bedside," European Heart Journal vol. 36, no. 48, (2015): pp. 3404-3412.

CHAPTER 20: MOTIVATION: DIVINE TREASURE

The study of the International Agency for Research on Cancer, based on data from Eastern Europe on a **smoker's risk of developing cancer**: Brennan, P., et al., "High Cumulative Risk of Lung Cancer Death Among Smokers and Nonsmokers in Central and Eastern Europe," *American Journal of Epidemiology* vol. 164, no. 12, (2006): pp. 1233-1241.

The study on the **risk of lung cancer in smokers in Canada** is in Villeneuve, P. J., and Mao, Y., "Lifetime Probability of Developing Lung Cancer, by Smoking Status," *Canadian Journal of Public Health* vol. 85, no. 6, (1994): pp. 385-388.

The Harvard School of Public Health study that analyzed the **premature deaths from smoking in women** is Kenfield, S., et al., "Smoking and Smoking Cessation in Relation to Mortality in Women," *JAMA* vol. 299, no. 17, (2008): pp. 2037-2047.

The study that calculated the **years of life lost in the male and female population because of tobacco** is in Jha, P., et al., "21st-Century Hazards of Smoking and Benefits of Smoking Cessation in the United States," *The New England Journal of Medicine* vol. 368, no. 4, (2013): pp. 341-350.

The more complete analysis of the **years of life and quality of life lost by premature deaths and illnesses worldwide**: Global Burden of Disease Study 2013 Collaborators, "Global, Regional, and National Incidence, Prevalence, and Years Lived with Disability for Acute and Chronic Diseases 301 and Injuries in 188 Countries, 1990-2013: A Systematic Analysis for the Global Burden of Disease Study 2013," *The Lancet* vol. 386, no. 9995, (2015): pp. 743-800.

A detailed analysis of the **years of life and quality of life lost in the population over 60** is in Prince, M. J., et al., "The Burden of Disease in Older People and Implications for Health Policy and Practice," *The Lancet* vol. 385, no. 9967, (2015): pp. 549-562.

An analysis of **the behavior and dietary habits that harm health** is located in Ezzati, M., and Riboli, E., "Behavioral and Dietary Risk Factors for Noncommunicable Disease," *The New England Journal of Medicine* vol. 369, no. 10, (2013): pp. 954-964.

CHAPTER 21: HOW LONG DO WE WANT TO LIVE?

The **challenge of increasing longevity** of the population on a global scale is discussed in Beard, J., et al., "The World Report on Ageing and Health: A Policy Framework for Healthy Ageing," *The Lancet* vol. 387, no. 10033, (2016): pp. 2145-2154.

The case of **Japan as a model society of great longevity** explained in Akiyama, H., "Japan's Longevity Challenge," *Science* vol. 350, no. 6265, (2015): p. 1135. And also McCurry, J., "Japan Will Be Model for Future Super-Aging Societies," *The Lancet* vol. 386, no. 10003, (2015): pp. 1523.

ABOUT THE AUTHORS

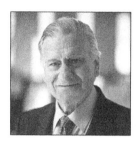 **VALENTIN FUSTER** serves Mount Sinai Hospital as physician-in-chief, as well as director of Mount Sinai Heart, and he is the general director of the National Center for Cardiovascular Investigation in Madrid, Spain. He has taught at numerous universities, held innumerable positions, and won many of the highest awards for his research. Dr. Fuster's work was the focus of the 2017 documentary *The Resilient Heart*.

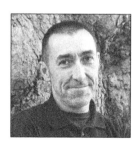 **JOSEP CORBELLA** is a Spanish journalist focusing on biomedicine and human evolution. Together with Valentin Fuster, he has written *The Heart Manual* (2006) and *Cooking for Health* (2010, also cowritten by Ferran Adrià). He has also published *The Wonderful Story of Your Body* (2018) and coauthored *Sapiens* (2000).